Chicken Soup for the Soul
Healthy Living:
Diabetes

Jack Canfield

Mark Victor Hansen

Byron Hoogwerf, M.D.
THE CLEVELAND CLINIC

Health Communications, Inc.
Deerfield Beach, Florida

www.bcibooks.com
www.chickensoup.com

We would like to acknowledge the many publishers and individuals who granted us permission to reprint the cited material.

I Can't Do It. Reprinted by permission of Page Garfinkel. ©2005 Page Garfinkel.

A Medal-Winning Diabetes Support Team. Reprinted by permission of Gary Hall. ©2005 Gary μHall.

The Gift. Reprinted by permission of Sally Friedman. ©2004 Sally Friedman.

My Wake-Up Call. Reprinted by permission of Dvora Waysman. ©2005 Dvora Waysman.

(Continued on page 133)

Library of Congress Cataloging-in-Publication Data

Diabetes / [edited by] Jack Canfield, Mark Victor Hansen, Byron Hoogwerf.
    p. cm. — (Chicken soup for the soul healthy living)
ISBN 0-7573-0488-5

    1. Diabetes—Popular works. I. Title: At head of title: Chicken soup for the soul healthy living. II. Canfield, Jack, 1944–
III. Hansen, Mark Victor. IV. Hoogwerf, Byron. V. Chicken soup for the soul healthy living series.

    RC660.4.D48 2006
    616.4'62—dc22

                    2005-56036

Publisher: Health Communications, Inc.
          3201 S.W. 15th Street
          Deerfield Beach, FL 33442–8190

Cover design by Larissa Hise Henoch
Inside book design by Lawna Patterson Oldfield

Fear less, hope more,

eat less, chew more,

whine less, breathe more,

talk less, say more,

love more,

and all good things

will be yours.

—Swedish Proverb

Contents

Introduction

"**Y**ou have diabetes." Just three little words, but together they form a very powerful sentence. And no matter how many times I have delivered that news to patients, I can never be sure of the exact response.

A diagnosis of diabetes can be a big shock. Rightly so, because diabetes is a serious medical condition. After hearing the news, many patients go through a series of several emotions—often including anger, denial, sadness and sometimes even depression.

Fortunately, most patients soon learn to accept their diagnosis and adapt the rigors of diabetes management into their lifestyle, at least for the most part. I will not go so far as to say a patient should jump for joy after learning they have diabetes, but there are ways to make lemonade when life hands you this bowl of lemons.

The best case scenario? You will recognize this diagnosis as a wake-up call that you have been lax in maintaining an optimal healthy lifestyle. You will use the diagnosis of diabetes as motivation to embark on a totally new approach to healthy living.

If you are lucky—and dedicated enough to stick to your new healthier lifestyle—you may even be able to reduce, delay or even avoid the need for medications.

However, sometimes medication is a necessary fact of life for people with diabetes. But equally as important as anything that comes in a pill or needle are other "treatments" such as keeping a good attitude and benefiting from a strong support system.

You probably have many questions about diabetes, and hopefully I will answer most of them in this book. Perhaps more important, I hope the diabetes experiences shared by contributors will inspire and enlighten you—and, in some cases, give you a much-needed chuckle.

I leave you with this final thought: Even the best medical treatment will only have limited success if you don't nurture your inner self and emotional health at the same time.

Wishing you a healthy and happy life, with or without diabetes.

♥ Byron Hoogwerf, M.D.
The Cleveland Clinic

I Can't Do It

"I can't do it," Adrian blurted as I started to explain how to count carbohydrates to control his blood sugar levels. "I have to give myself four injections and check my blood sugar ten times a day and now you want me to count how many grams of carbohydrates I am supposed to eat as well? I just want to have fun like all of my friends and not think about so many things. I see what happens to people who get diabetes. Why should I even bother?" Adrian looked beaten. Being alive had become a chore that he wasn't very enthusiastic about fulfilling.

At eighteen years old, Adrian had many psychological issues to deal with regarding his diabetes. He was too young to be so accountable for his health. Adrian had many considerations; he needed to follow a schedule—a demanding schedule. His friends didn't share this level of responsibility at all. "Adrian, let me tell you a little story," I said, hoping that I could help to change his perspective about his disease. I wanted him to realize that less than a century ago he would have died.

"You see, Adrian," I said as I began my story, "before 1922, children were starving to death from diabetes. Without insulin, these kids couldn't feed their body with energy or sugar and the body would literally eat itself to death. James Havens, the son of the vice president of Eastman Kodak, was the first child to be treated with insulin in the United States. His weight was down to seventy-three pounds and he was dying. Insulin saved his life. Five-year-old Teddy Ryder was down to twenty-seven pounds and approaching death when he received insulin and went on to live until he was seventy-six years old. Then there was Elizabeth Hughes, the daughter of United States Secretary of State Charles Evans Hughes. Diabetes ravaged her body until her weight was below forty-five pounds and she could barely walk. Her doctor put her on a starvation diet to prolong her life. It allowed her to live long enough for a treatment to be discovered. Within weeks of the discovery of insulin and her visit to Dr. Banting in Toronto, she began gaining weight and her health improved significantly in no time. Elizabeth went on to marry and have children. She died at age seventy-three.

"Eighty years ago, you would not have lived unless you were one of the fortunate ones who survived long enough for insulin to be discovered. For you, Adrian, there is a long and healthy road ahead if you care to follow it. I will give you the tools to save your own life and then it's up to you."

Adrian sat still in contemplation about his disease, his life and the choices he was forced to make. "Twenty-seven pounds and forty-five pounds? How could they have lived?" Adrian asked, looking overwhelmed at how destructive "his" disease could be.

"As humans, we want to survive. We fight until the end. Their fight was painful, uncontrollable and horribly scary. All they were able to do was pray that a treatment or cure would be found before their bodies gave up," I said. "And for *some* their prayers were answered."

"I suppose these children were so thankful to be alive that they were grateful to follow a regimented treatment plan," Adrian said, realizing how truly fortunate he was. "So, did you say I need to inject five units of insulin for my breakfast?"

"Yes, and if you would like I can give you other breakfast samples and we can figure out how much insulin will be needed. And you know what? I bet a cure is within reach. Maybe you can join me in the Walk to Cure Diabetes next Saturday?"

"I'll be there!" Adrian smiled as our session ended. His new outlook on life was just beginning.

♥ *Page Garfinkel*

A Medal-Winning
Diabetes Support Team

I had spent my entire life eating right, exercising
and minding my health. Something like this
wasn't supposed to happen to someone like me. I was
an Olympic swimmer, a world class athlete. But in
1999, I started experiencing a number of symptoms,
like blurred vision, constant fatigue and an unquench-
able thirst. Finally, after collapsing at a party, I was
diagnosed with Type 1 diabetes at the age of 25.

As most people with diabetes will tell you, taking
the first decisive step to admit you need help isn't
easy; some would argue that it's the hardest step in
the diabetes care process. I'm here to tell you that it
isn't any easier when your doctors are telling you that
you won't ever be able to do the one thing you've
been training for throughout your whole life.   I was
a week away from the Spring Nationals and had been
feeling more confident in my swimming, but all of a
sudden I felt like my whole world was crashing down
around me. My girlfriend at the time—now my
wife—became my support system. She stuck by my

side even when I felt like giving up completely, and she encouraged me when I wasn't sure if I would ever swim competitively again. I was lucky.

As an Olympic athlete, I was used to being surrounded by a team of people who would work with me to help me train and achieve my goals. After thorough research, I was able to add diabetes experts to my team of coaches. I surrounded myself with a team of experts from across the country who believed that I would continue to swim and who knew I could go for the gold despite my diabetes. They helped me learn how to care for myself; how to monitor my blood glucose levels to avoid getting too high or too low, how and when to inject my insulin—my life line. Essentially, I had to relearn how to live my life to incorporate my diabetes care needs.

Not everyone is so lucky. I have been very active in the diabetes community since I was diagnosed, and I often meet people who feel alone in their challenge to manage their disease. I was fortunate enough to meet a few people who reminded me how lucky I was when I became involved in the BD Diabetes Makeover program. The participants in the Makeover program came together from all over the country to get a better grip on their diabetes management. Like so many others, they had lost the motivation somewhere in a busy, often hectic life to give their diabetes the attention it needed. Some didn't have access to the right tools and information. For others, the mention of diabetes was met with a groan, and a mental acknowledgment that they needed to start monitoring their diabetes in a more aggressive way to get their blood glucose level back where it belonged.

When I first met the Makeover participants, I was immediately overwhelmed by their enthusiasm. The teamwork they demonstrated reminded me of the team attitude I was accustomed to at the Olympic level. Everyone, including Olympic athletes, needs encouragement and support—and the room was full of it. They became my inspiration, despite the fact that I was there to be theirs. The determination I saw in their eyes, and seeing these ordinary people take control of their lives, motivates me to test my blood glucose levels when I don't feel like it, to give myself that extra shot of insulin, and to swim an extra lap in training.

The team approach paid off for those participants just as it paid off for me. I managed to win four more medals in the 2000 Olympics, as well as two more in 2004. But those medals belong not only to me, not only to my team of coaches and doctors, but to everyone out there who is determined to control their diabetes and take charge of their lives.

♥ Gary Hall Jr., 10-time Olympic medalist in swimming

A Wake-Up Call

Diabetes is a disease that causes the body to not produce enough insulin, or not use it properly. Insulin is essential to keep your body functioning properly.

This is a serious disease that should not be taken lightly. For many people, the diagnosis can actually end up having a positive effect, because it gives them a much-needed wake-up call to make some important changes in their life, and their lifestyle.

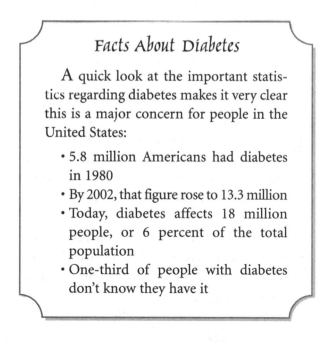

Facts About Diabetes

A quick look at the important statistics regarding diabetes makes it very clear this is a major concern for people in the United States:

- 5.8 million Americans had diabetes in 1980
- By 2002, that figure rose to 13.3 million
- Today, diabetes affects 18 million people, or 6 percent of the total population
- One-third of people with diabetes don't know they have it

Think about . . .
what diabetes means to me

- What (if any) serious symptoms and complications do I need to address right away?

- What lifestyle changes can I make immediately?

- Do I need insulin, pills or other regular treatment? If so, how can I incorporate that into my daily schedule?

- Do I need to find a medical specialist?

- How can I best benefit from the help of friends and family?

- Where can I find a good support system?

- How am I going to change my lifestyle in the long term to improve my health?

And, perhaps most important:

- How can I put a positive spin on this, and maintain a good attitude?

The Gift

I t was a particularly beautiful spring day when I went to my gynecologist for a routine checkup and held out my finger for a needle prick. It was the first time that office had asked for a small blood sample, an acknowledgment that a gynecologist is often the only doctor many women see.

I was feeling on top of the world that day. Midlife was turning out to be a time of freedom, growth and terrific well-being. I hadn't even had a cold in months. My weight was fine. What did I have to worry about?

"Your blood sugar is extremely high," my gynecologist announced unceremoniously. "What did you eat before you came here?"

I recounted my sin almost jauntily, still not getting it. Lunch had been the usual: a fat bagel and a Reese's Peanut Butter Cup, my daily indulgence. Dr. J. didn't smile. In fact, she looked rather grim as she advised me to get to an endocrinologist immediately. My reading at her office had grazed 300. A normal blood glucose one hour after eating, I would later learn, would have been far lower, probably in the range of 120 to 140.

The endocrinologist tested me again, and again found higher than normal readings. Talk about wake-up calls . . .

I've had a lifelong obsession with weight. As a formerly chubby child, I'd vowed never to be anything but slim, so I'd leaped into the dangerous waters of crazy eating. To satisfy both the obsession—and the sweet tooth—I'd practically lived my adult life on limited doses of candy bars, cookies and an occasional protein. It's a wonder I'd made it without incident as long as I had.

Ah, but people admired my slimness—and that was the dubious reward for such self-punishing eating habits. I grooved on sliding into a size eight for decades.

Suddenly, however, I was no longer just a woman with a sweet tooth. I was prediabetic. And that made my self-imposed dietary route to size eight feel utterly foolish and yes, dangerous.

Life is definitely different now. I have a new and intense awareness of the importance of diet and exercise in my life, and I take it seriously. It took months, even years, for me to learn to relish foods that would love me back. But today, I'm as excited—well, almost—about devouring a huge, healthful salad as I was with the chocolate chip cookies of yore.

I'm also the proud owner of a home testing kit that allows me to check and monitor my blood sugars regularly. And as a former confirmed coward who practically fainted at the sight of a needle, I'm pleased to report that I do my finger sticks without even flinching. I know how important the monitoring is.

What still haunts me is that I didn't have a single symptom. That realization is also what keeps me committed to working hard to avoid what I have come to think of as falling off the looming cliff: developing full-blown diabetes.

So far, it's working. So far, my blood sugars are squarely in the normal range, which is where they have remained since May of 1994.

And what's happened to my proud size eight status? It's changed. Given my new healthy eating, and an exercise regimen that includes nightly walks with my husband during which we solve the world's problems, I'm now a size six.

Am I perfect at sticking to the healthy life? Of course not. There are still times when a peanut butter cup solves more emotional problems than a carrot stick. I keep the peanut butter cups in the freezer, however, and buy them on a one-at-a-time basis to make access a bit harder.

On our refrigerator door is a little yellowing piece of paper. It's the original note from my gynecologist, ominous blood sugar numbers boldly scrawled in her semi-indecipherable handwriting.

It will always remind me of the "gift" of that long-ago finger prick, and how it changed my life. In real and symbolic terms, that little drop of blood may even have saved it.

♥ *Sally Friedman*

The Diagnosis

It's relatively easy to diagnose diabetes. Here's the typical process:

- Symptoms indicate possibility of diabetes
- Initial blood test to check sugar levels
- Fasting plasma glucose test
- Urine test to check sugar and ketone levels

TYPE 1 DIABETES

If you are diagnosed with diabetes, you will fall into one of two categories. The first, Type 1 diabetes, involves a failure to produce insulin.

- Previously called juvenile diabetes, this type of diabetes is often diagnosed during childhood (according to the American Diabetes Association, about one in every 400 to 500 children and teens have it).
- While commonly detected during childhood, it can develop at any age.
- Although the exact cause of Type 1 diabetes is unknown, it is an "autoimmune" disease in which antibodies damage the insulin-producing cells.
- There is no vaccine for diabetes, and no way to prevent it, at least in the case of Type 1 diabetes.

TYPE 2 DIABETES

- The majority of people with diabetes have Type 2 diabetes.
- Doctors haven't yet figured out exactly what causes this type of diabetes, but people with a family history of the disease do seem to be at higher risk.
- Unlike people with Type 1 diabetes, people with Type 2 diabetes do produce insulin. They just aren't producing enough of it, or it's not being used as it should. This involves insulin resistance—in other words, the body isn't using insulin properly.
- Most people with Type 2 diabetes are overweight.

On a positive note, it is preventable in many cases. Preventative steps include:

- Watching your weight
- Following a sensible diet
- Exercising regularly (at least 150 minutes per week minimum)

What Is Insulin, Anyway?

You can't talk about diabetes without discussing insulin. What is insulin, exactly? Insulin is a hormone produced by the body. Its job is to deliver nutrients—especially glucose—into cells in various parts of the body. Remember how glucose travels through your body through the metabolism process? Well, it can't get into many cells by itself. It needs insulin to help carry it into muscle cells for energy or fat cells for storage. Insulin generally goes to work after you eat. If you eat something that's high in sugar, your body will need a lot of insulin to handle this.

Could You Have Diabetes?

Many people with diabetes do not have any obvious symptoms. If someone you love has diabetes, now is a good time to think about having yourself checked as well. Here are some common symptoms that are often a telltale sign of diabetes:

- Always feeling thirsty, especially when accompanied by frequent urination
- Losing weight
- Constantly feeling tired

Risk factors include:

- Family history
- Weight problems
- High blood pressure
- Sedentary lifestyle
- Age
- Ethnic background (Hispanics, Native Americans and African Americans have a higher risk)

If you have any of the symptoms, or any other signs that you suspect may signal diabetes, see your doctor right away.

⚕ *Think about . . .*
things to ask my doctor

- What type of diabetes do I have?

- How high are my sugar levels?

- What treatment plan do you recommend?

- Why are you giving me this type of medicine? What does it do? What are possible side effects?

- Can you give me a good diet plan, or recommend a nutritionist who can?

- Are any of my vital signs or lab results (cholesterol level, blood pressure, weight, etc.) a cause for concern?

My Wake-Up Call

Diabetes, like life, is something that happened to me when I wasn't looking. I may have been walking around with this disease for years without knowing it, because I had none of the classic symptoms you read about, like a raging thirst. In fact I felt great, despite knowing at some level that I was genetically disposed to Type 2 (adult onset) diabetes. But like the old motto says—"If it ain't broke, don't fix it"—I didn't think about being tested. Why go looking for trouble?

Then one day, about ten years ago, there was a leaflet in my letter box announcing a Health Fair in the suburb where I live. I now think of it as the luckiest day of my life, because I am sure that if I hadn't bothered to walk over to the local Community Center, I wouldn't be alive today.

I went more out of curiosity than anything else. Lots of tables were set out on the grounds, manned by doctors, and you could be tested free for a whole range of illnesses. I had planned to go to the blood pressure testing but the line was too long and I had no patience. There was nobody at the diabetes testing table, so I sat down and agreed to be tested.

The doctor asked me to fill out a medical history and, upon seeing my family history of diabetes, seemed astonished that I had never checked it out before. She took a drop of blood from my finger, placed it on a test strip and measured my blood glucose level. I saw her face go ashen as the result showed a reading of 375. It didn't mean anything to me. Then she tested me again, with the same result.

"I think I should call an ambulance," she said. "You must go to the hospital."

I laughed and told her I'd never felt better. But after she talked to me seriously for a few minutes, I realized it was no laughing matter. I was a serious diabetic, and a candidate for heart disease, kidney disease, blindness, limb amputation and premature death. I didn't want to go to the hospital, but promised to consult a doctor the next day and make any lifestyle changes necessary to bring the glucose level down.

So, at age sixty, I began to live sensibly (well, I'm a slow learner!). I had always had a love affair with food, especially cakes, ice cream and chocolate. I didn't go on a crash diet or one that made me feel continually deprived, but I thought about everything I put in my mouth. I made choices. Lots of salads and a piece of fruit when I needed something

sweet. Lower fat, achieved by buying 1% milk
instead of 3%, and yogurt and cottage cheese with
no fat. High fiber breakfasts with porridge made
from oatmeal, and lots of oat bran. A few nuts.
Chicken and fish mostly replacing red meat.
Cooking creatively, using dates, raisins or small
amounts of artificial sweeteners when necessary.

The dietary changes had to be accompanied by
exercise, and at first this was difficult for me. Up
until then, my most strenuous exercise was playing
Scrabble. But now I leave home at 6 A.M. each week-
day morning, and speed walk for at least forty minutes. Gradually, I've grown to enjoy it. The
traffic-free air is pure at that time, and the only
sounds are birdsongs. Most mornings you meet the
same people, walkers like yourself, a few joggers,
people walking their dogs. You don't talk but you
smile at each other as you pass. You understand
each other. In winter it's harder but if you dress
appropriately it's still possible, although often it's
dark when I leave home. If it's raining heavily, I use
my exercise bicycle and I work out at home.

Paradoxical as it sounds, diabetes has enabled me
to appreciate life so much more. There are things I
want to do including writing more books and danc-
ing at the weddings of our eighteen lovely grandchildren. I try to remember a saying I read many
years ago. There is a beautiful Chinese home in the

heart of Peking. The garden is enclosed by a high wall, and on one side, surrounded by twining red and white flowers, there is a brass plate about two feet long. The inscription has changed many people's lives. Translated, it reads: "Enjoy yourself. It is later than you think!"

♥ *Dvora Waysman*

Putting a Positive Spin on Your Diagnosis

It's easy to have an instinctive negative reaction after hearing a diabetes diagnosis. But once you get over the initial shock, you can often turn this around into a good thing by viewing the diagnosis as a wake-up call that prompts you to realize how valuable your health is and adopt better lifestyle habits. That's not all—there are many other ways to put a positive spin on this diagnosis:

Scout out the best fitness club in town, and encourage friends to join you in group workouts. No fitness facilities in town? Take action and see if you can help bring one to the area.

Sign up for a 5K race—or a walkathon if that's more your speed—and encourage people to join you. Or participate in a charity event and ask people to sponsor you. You'll get exercise while raising money for a good cause.

Search out the best biking or hiking trails in your community. If you don't have any, lobby your local government to establish some.

Spend some extra time with a good friend by walking or biking together regularly.

Volunteer to speak at local schools or community organizations, sharing your knowledge on diabetes and tips for avoiding the disease.

MAINTAIN A HEALTHY SENSE OF HUMOR

Sure, a diabetes diagnosis may be serious, but that doesn't mean you have to be, at least not all the time. They say laughter is good for the soul, so think of this as doctor's orders: Try to find the humor in life as much as possible.

> Inform your friends that part of your new mandated exercise routine will include *skipping* household chores, *dodging* telemarketers, *running* up your credit card balances—and, oh yeah, *chasing* your dreams.
>
> Announce that you can never *eat* your words, *swallow* your pride or *taste* defeat—because you don't know their carb counts.
>
> Compete with friends and family to see who can come up with the corniest diabetes joke.

KEEP A POSITIVE OUTLOOK!

Of course, like any wake-up call, this is one you might not be thrilled to get. And nobody expects you to jump for joy yelling, "Hooray! I just found out I've got diabetes!" But it *is* important to stay positive and try to look on the bright side.

Ideally, you've found out you have diabetes before experiencing any serious problems. If so, count your blessings. And therein lies the true gift of diabetes—it forces you to treasure your life, and your health, and to start taking steps to protect them both.

As with any medical issue, your outlook regarding diabetes can greatly affect how you feel physically. So if you stay positive and stay motivated about sticking with healthy lifestyle changes, you will probably keep yourself physically healthier.

Together Forever

Gertrude Samuels came in with her husband, Harry, for her first diabetes education session when she was eighty-seven years old. "Gertrude, I'm going to give you a meal plan and explain why it's important to make healthy food choices," I said, hoping she would be willing to control this disease even at her advanced age. Some of my younger patients felt that it infringed on their lives and virtually ignored their condition.

"Marci, you tell me what to do and I will do it!" Gertrude said with a serious tone.

"I have diabetes too, and we need to take care of each other," a timid Harry Samuels added. Harry looked to be about his wife's age. "We've been married for sixty-five years. We do everything together—even get diabetes!"

Harry, like Gertrude, had a slight build. He sat close to his wife and touched her arm gently as he spoke. "I've tested her blood sugar and it runs high and low, high and low. I just don't know what to do." Harry looked worried.

"That's why you're here. By the time you leave my office you will know exactly what you need to do. Can I take your blood sugar now, Gertrude?" I asked, hoping to see how her breakfast meal affected her reading.

"Surely." Gertrude held out her hand. I cleaned her finger with alcohol and dried it with a gauze pad and then I took a small sample of blood from her middle finger. The results came five seconds later and read 38 mg/dl (milligrams per deciliter).

"Thirty-eight! You've got extremely low blood sugar. How do you feel?" I was shocked that her blood sugar was so far below 70; the more typical low blood sugar level.

"I feel just fine," Gertrude stated honestly.

"Let me double-check this reading with another machine just in case." I hurriedly grabbed another machine and it was indeed correct. "Yes, it's 38 mg/dl. Well, let me get you some juice before your blood sugar gets any lower and you pass out on me!" I stepped out of my office and literally ran to the refrigerator to get a large glass of juice and some cheese and crackers. "Here you go. Please drink this juice and then we will re-test the blood sugar and see if it gets up to at least 100."

Gertrude drank her juice and fifteen minutes later her blood sugar went up to 124 mg/dl. "Okay, now you can eat these crackers and cheese, if you don't mind. We don't want your blood sugar to drop back down again and that can happen unless you eat something more substantial. Protein helps you digest your food more slowly so if you combine the cheese with carbohydrates (crackers, for example) then you will maintain a level blood sugar." I felt more comfortable with this new reading and confident that she wouldn't get that awful low blood sugar. "We'll just check it one more time before you leave to be absolutely sure you are okay."

During the next five years I thought about them at times. I thought about being in love with the same person for sixty-five years, having had children, grandchildren and great-grandchildren and how lucky and comforting it must be to have the same person by your side as long as you or they would live. Then, I thought of the inconceivable devastation one must feel to lose their lifelong partner whom they spent most of their years with.

One morning my phone rang at work. "Marci, this is Gertrude Samuels, how are you?"

"Fine!" I said, so very pleased to hear her voice. "And how are you and your husband?" I hesitantly asked. After all, it was five years later and they were now ninety-two years plus.

"We're both great! Can I ask you a question?"

"Of course, what can I help you with?" I asked

feeling somewhat emotional that she and Harry were alive and well.

"I wanted to buy one of those new blood sugar monitors I saw advertised that need a tiny bit of blood. Which one would you recommend?" Gertrude sounded strong, healthy and happy. I couldn't get over it. I was thrilled to have been able to give them the knowledge to control their diabetes and that they chose to use it. I was more than impressed that these two lovebirds wanted an updated blood sugar monitor to use. "Why don't you come in for a quick hello and I'll give you a monitor—my favorite one—and I'll show you how to use it as well. I'd love to see you both." I wanted the chance to see my favorite couple; both with diabetes, married for seventy years now, and still going strong.

"You're so sweet, what time would be good?" Gertrude hadn't changed.

The next day Gertrude and Harry Samuels came into my office. They looked the same. I showed them how to use their new blood sugar monitor and quickly checked their blood sugar. "105 for you, Gertrude, and 106 for you, Harry, and that was after eating the same breakfast I recommended over five years ago: oatmeal, blueberries, cinnamon and chopped walnuts. Excellent, great job! Keep up the good work." Apparently, they had followed my diet recommendations to the letter.

"We couldn't have stayed so healthy without the knowledge you provided us with. You saved my wife and because of that you saved me too," Harry said as tears welled up in his eyes.

As they walked out the door I thought, *May they live at least as many years as their blood sugar readings that morning.*

♥ *Marci Sloane*

A *Diagnosis of Diabetes*

Two years ago my husband was rushed to the hospital because he could not breathe and had severe pain in his chest and back, along with a cold sweat. We assumed it was respiratory in nature, as he had a history of chronic bronchitis and he recently suffered what we thought was an asthma attack while hiking in our local mountains.

I followed about fifteen minutes behind the ambulance, and arrived in the emergency room rather shocked and winded. He was only thirty-seven, and though he had a few minor health problems, he was in relatively good shape. I quickly made my way through the halls to his side. He looked okay—sitting upright, rather shocked himself but in a good state of mind overall. He has the graceful ability to smile and laugh through challenge. The ER doctor explained that my husband had either a collapsed lung or pneumonia. I nodded my head, as if agreeing with his diagnosis, internally trying as hard as I could to remain calm.

At the same time, we learned my husband was

diabetic. Upon his arrival in the ER, they had tested his blood sugar. When the doctor had told him, rather animatedly, "Your blood sugar is over 400!," my husband had simply said, "Okay . . ." Perplexed by his rather nonchalant response, the doctor then asked when he had been diagnosed with diabetes. It was, of course, news to him that he had diabetes. But, compared to the other diagnoses, a collapsed lung or pneumonia, it really didn't register as being a very big deal.

After a week in the hospital, it became clear that his situation wasn't improving and he was transferred to a larger hospital that was much better equipped for more complicated cases of pneumonia. There we found out that he had a serious lung infection, which had indeed resulted in a collapsed lung. It was a long and exhausting two weeks, as he received strong antibiotics and several procedures—including major surgery—to overcome the illness. During this time we met with diabetes educators. It all seemed like Greek to us—the idea of keeping track not only of blood sugar, but also of carbohydrate intake, new medications, and for the first few months, insulin! I learned as much as I could about his situation, practiced giving shots, and even—at the coaxing of an educator—gave myself a "shot" with an empty syringe.

Leaving the hospital, we felt overwhelmed. Not

only did he have several months of recovery ahead
of him (which entailed a portable antibiotic IV and
the healing of a rib that had been broken during
surgery), he also had to learn how to live as someone with diabetes. This meant a complete assess-
ment of his diet, a cleaning out of the pantry, a
quick collection of low-carbohydrate recipes,
blood-sugar testing five times each day, and regular
injections. Because he had Type 2 diabetes, it was
not expected he would remain on insulin once his
blood sugar was under control, so sudden episodes
of hypoglycemia were a concern as well.

Slowly, as his body healed from the surgery, he
began walking and lifting very light free weights. He
had lost about thirty pounds in the hospital and
soon gained back a healthy amount of weight in
muscle. His cholesterol dropped thirty points
through diet and exercise alone, and within only
three months his A1C went from over 12—as measured in the hospital—to 5.7. He soon became his
endocrinologist's dream patient, demonstrating that
a positive and informed approach to a new discovery of diabetes can have a terrific effect on physical
health. Indeed, his lifestyle changes have had a positive effect on the rest of our family as well.

It has now been two years since the diagnosis of
an illness that could have killed him. He sometimes
says it was the best thing that happened to him,

because it offered him the motivation to change poor lifestyle habits and get into the shape he is finally in, doing the active things he loves, and eating foods that make him feel great. And although he is certainly not happy to have diabetes, he welcomes its reminder to live well, and to enjoy the truly important things in life.

♥ *Nellie Levine*

The Sugar Story

To understand how diabetes affects your body, it's helpful to learn about your metabolism. Oh sure, many of us are familiar with the word—if our clothes suddenly get too tight, we blame our metabolism for being too slow.

Metabolism is actually the process in which your body uses food for energy. Your body is like a machine, and it needs fuel to keep running. That fuel comes in the form of the things you eat and drink. But your body's cells are very small and can't handle something like, say, a pizza with the works. That's why your organs need to digest the food and break it down into very tiny substances. This is metabolism at work.

SUGAR: IT ISN'T ALWAYS SO SWEET

One of these basic substances is glucose, which is a simple sugar. Glucose is transported to millions of cells throughout your entire body, where it helps provide the energy all your body parts need in order to keep working.

Glucose is either ingested through food or created by the body (in the liver, to be exact). It is then distributed to various cells in the body, to be either used immediately (by the muscles, for example) or stored as fat.

Sugar Substitutes

These days, it's easier than ever to reduce your sugar intake without feeling deprived. Sugar substitutes like Splenda and NutraSweet are used in many sugar-free products (that actually taste good!) and are also available in packets for using at home in drinks and baking. NutraSweet doesn't tend to work well for baking, though, so Splenda may be a better choice for that use.

Not Too Bad

"I t's not too bad . . ."

I smiled as my husband uttered the reluctant compliment. For years I had been trying to persuade him to change from drinking regular soda to diet soda, ever since the doctor first diagnosed his diabetes.

"It's not too bad . . ."

From entrees to desserts, we changed our menus and eating habits—except for soda. Diet soda became our line of demarcation. It represented the difference between two lifestyles: "normal" and "diabetic." No longer was food simply for nutritional benefit or enjoyment. Now it represented something ominous, even life-threatening. Every bite was regarded suspiciously as we became amateur sleuths searching for hidden traces of sneaky sugar.

"It's not too bad . . ."

Was life to become a series of "not-too-bad" experiences? We hoped not. There's something depressing about "not-too-bad." It carries a sad implication of compromise—of settling for second-best or third-rate. Nobody wants that. And yet, the alternative is so much worse.

We changed our eating habits, plunging into a world of sugar substitutes and low carbs. Except for the soda—the lone holdout in a sea of change. Until that one day . . .

"It's not too bad . . ."

The first sip is the hardest.

Of course, as with any change, we adapt and we adjust. Our taste buds are no different. What was once strange soon became familiar. What was familiar quickly became normal. And what was normal rapidly became flavorful.

Now the diet soda in the refrigerator is just another part of our routine. It reflects awareness that it's the little things that add up to a healthy lifestyle. Walking, exercising, eating right, getting enough sleep. They all work together for a good life—*our* good life. There's nothing second-best or third-rate about it, because it contributes to the health we enjoy each minute of every day.

"It's not too bad" never sounded so good.

♥ *Ava Pennington*

Expecting a Miracle

It wasn't fair. It just wasn't fair.

After two years of trying to conceive the doctor had finally coaxed my body into ovulating and now my husband and I were expecting our first child. We were ecstatic, eagerly preparing for the future.

Only now the doctor was telling me I had gestational diabetes.

I'd known I was high risk. Not only were both of my parents Type 2 diabetics, the condition behind my infertility was linked to hyperinsulinemia, a condition which caused my body to be unresponsive to insulin. Getting pregnant had required taking medicine for diabetes control as well as fertility drugs.

But it still didn't seem fair.

When I got home from the doctor's office I laid down on my bed and sobbed. My stupid body! I hated it. It wouldn't let me get pregnant without medical intervention and now it wouldn't let my baby grow in peace inside me. The doctor had been careful to impress me with the seriousness of the situation, filling my head with horror stories about babies grown too large, being delivered with dislocated shoulders or plunging blood sugar levels.

It seemed like my body was poisoning my precious baby and it broke my heart.

The next few months were spent thinking about food. I measured everything I ate, learned to ignore unapproved cravings, checked my blood sugar levels at least four times a day. Most of the time my levels were within the range my doctor had set for me, but there was one reading that just wouldn't come down. Every morning I'd check my blood before I ate breakfast, only to find that it was even higher before breakfast than it was two hours after eating.

Nothing the doctor and I tried could get that number down to where it should be. I tried eating something high protein just before bed. I tried getting up at two A.M. to have a snack. Still, morning after morning my blood sugar was over 100.

Finally the doctor put me on insulin. Just one shot, right before bedtime, only six units. "Don't worry," he told me. "We do this all the time. The baby will be perfectly safe."

Then he told me to come in for fetal monitoring twice a week for the rest of the pregnancy. I could also expect to be induced at 38 weeks, two weeks early. Just to be on the safe side.

I went home and cried some more.

At 37 weeks the doctor sent me for an ultrasound to determine the baby's size. To the amazement of my doctor and my intense joy, she was only a little over seven pounds. Not too small, not too large. It was as if I'd never had gestational diabetes at all.

In the end, the doctor let me go to a full 40 weeks. My daughter was eight and a half pounds when she was born, with no blood sugar or developmental problems.

This time my tears were for joy.

♥ *Jennifer Merrill*

Special Situations

PREDIABETES

Type 2 diabetes rarely crops up without warning. Most people who develop this disease go
through a "phasing in" period, where they are
heading toward diabetes but don't actually have it
yet. This is called prediabetes. The primary sign of
prediabetes: glucose levels are higher than the ideal
range, but not high enough to be considered in the
diabetic range.

The good news? If you act quickly at this stage,
you can often prevent Type 2 diabetes before it
starts. Simple changes like a healthier diet and better fitness routine can make a world of difference.

GESTATIONAL DIABETES

Pregnant women sometimes get gestational diabetes. This is a term used to refer to a condition in
which women who did not previously have diabetes
suddenly exhibit high glucose levels.

- It's not totally clear what causes some women
  to develop this condition, but some risk factors
  may include being overweight, over age twenty-
  five or of an ethnic group with a high incidence
  of diabetes.

- It usually develops late in pregnancy and can be harmful to mother and baby.
- Diet adjustments and increased activity often help, but insulin treatment may sometimes be necessary.

⚕ Think about . . .
a prediabetes diagnosis

- How I feel about having prediabetes: _____

  _____

  _____

- What I have done to educate myself about diabetes: _____

  _____

  _____

- Improvements I have made to my fitness level:

  _____

  _____

  _____

- Positive changes I have made to my diet: _____

  _____

  _____

- Other lifestyle changes I've made to avoid getting diabetes: _____

  _____

  _____

- People I have enlisted to be part of my support team: _____

  _____

The Diabetes Boat

My doctor opened the thick file and nodded a few times. Then she looked up at me. "Okay, Harriet," she said. "Which do you want first? The good news or the bad news?"

I thought for a minute and the pessimist side of me won out. "The bad news."

"You have prediabetes."

I gulped. Not that I was surprised, but even a pessimist can be a closet optimist. "What's the good news? I have a year to live?"

"No," she said. "The good news is that if you start taking better care of yourself right now, you may never develop full-blown diabetes. You could live to be a hundred." She tapped her fingers on the file. "You already have hypothyroidism and arthritis. Both of those conditions put you at a higher risk of getting diabetes. As for your weight . . ." Her voice trailed off.

I tugged at my blouse and instinctively sucked in my stomach. For a second, my waistband relaxed but as soon as I took another breath, it stretched tight. My weight. I had been a "healthy" baby, a euphemism for fat. From there, I graduated to being a chubby child, a chunky teenager and an overweight adult. Now it looked as if I was going to add diabetic to the list of adjectives.

I slumped in my seat.

"Harriet, it's not the end of the world. Over 16 million North Americans are prediabetic."

"Well, at least I won't be alone in that sinking ship," I responded. When I looked in a mirror, I saw a middle-age woman who had a lifetime love affair with food and whose body had lost the fight with gravity. When I looked at my doctor, I saw a woman in her early thirties who probably didn't even know the meaning of cellulite. What I really needed, I decided, was a fat doctor who could empathize with me.

When I didn't respond, my doctor continued. "It's your choice. You can either lose weight and begin a regular exercise program, or you can start thinking about a future as an insulin-injecting diabetic person."

I wasn't sure who I disliked more at that moment—myself for being fat or my doctor for being thin. Thin and mean, I amended.

She spent the next fifteen minutes talking to me, but I only heard snatches of what she said. I must have nodded at the appropriate times because I left the office with a bunch of brochures clutched in my hands and a follow-up appointment.

Back on the street, I jammed the brochures into my purse and stopped at a local coffee shop. I ordered a coffee and a large bran muffin, telling myself that something filled with fiber must be good for me.

As I munched away, I looked around at the other occupants of the coffee shop. I mentally weighed each person, wondering which ones would end up in the sinking ship with me. The skinny girl with the blonde hair? The harried-looking plump mother with two toddlers? The overweight man reading a newspaper? Maybe all three of them, in which case I'd need a bigger boat.

I popped the last bite in my mouth and headed home.

For the next two weeks I continued to eat my favorite foods. *Better eat them while you still have a chance,* I told myself. In fact, have an extra piece of cake. Once you're diabetic, they'll all be forbidden.

But under the voice that told me to indulge lay another little voice that sounded suspiciously like my doctor's. *It's your choice,* the voice whispered as I wolfed down a generous helping of double fudge cake. *It's your choice,* it murmured as I savored a large baked potato dripping in sour cream. *It's your*

choice, it muttered as I reached for a second helping of pasta.

Although I tried to drown out the second voice
in food, it persisted.

"All right," I yelled one day. "Enough is enough.
You win. I'll give it a try. No more cake. No more
pasta. No more potatoes."

For the next two weeks I cut out cake, bread,
pasta and potatoes. And I was miserable. And hun-
gry. I snapped at everyone and everything. Even
though my pants zipped up without protest, I felt
too wretched to care.

I was cleaning out my purse the other day when
I found the diabetes brochures. I figured I'd read
them—anything to keep my mind off food. Halfway
through I realized that choice didn't have to mean
hunger. Choice meant selecting more nutritious
foods and smaller portions. It didn't mean that
bread, cake and pasta were banned—we just
couldn't be best friends anymore.

As I chewed on these new thoughts, I realized the
diabetes boat had turned into a life raft. This time
when I heard the little voice in my head, it chuckled.

♥ *Harriet Cooper*

Learn to Relax

As with any medical condition, stress can trigger an increase in side effects and complications—and can make it tougher for your body to perform at peak level. It's not always easy to relax, especially if you have a medical condition like diabetes and are trying to juggle all the issues and responsibilities that go along with it.

But it is vital that you give your body—and your mind—a break from stress and worry. Unfortunately, relaxing is often easier said than done. This doesn't come naturally to everyone, especially if you're born with a Type-A personality.

Luckily, there are ways to "train" yourself into making relaxing a part of your regular routine. Caution: once you start learning to relax, you may start wanting to do it a bit *too* much.

Enlist high-tech help. These days, there are many modern tools to help you relax. Try putting some classical music on your CD or MP3 player (be sure to use the headphones, to block out any distracting or stressful noise around you). Some people find it soothing to play a "white noise" machine—in a pinch, an air conditioner or fan that provides a similar noise can also do the trick. In addition, there are many relaxation tapes and CDs available, many of which feature the calming sounds of birds, waterfalls or other relaxing noises.

Try new age techniques. With today's fast-paced lifestyle, relaxation is a must for many people. There are many "new age" options available, including relaxation spas and retreats, yoga and Pilates classes, lots of different types of massages and meditation. Search your newspaper or look online for available resources in your area, or head to a major bookstore, where you'll find tons of books on all kinds of relaxation techniques.

Go old school. If you don't want anything complicated, high-tech or expensive, you can always employ basic old-fashioned relaxation strategies. Go for a walk in a quiet neighborhood, spend some time reading in the park or stake out a peaceful spot on the beach. Want to relax without leaving home? Stake out a quiet room or area of your home, and declare it off-limits to everyone else. Hopefully you can find an area that's as far as possible from the main hub of household activity—and if your hideaway spot has any kind of soundproof element, you've really hit the jackpot. Let everyone know you are not to be disturbed except for emergencies, and just enjoy the peace and quiet. For added relaxation, let your dog sit on your lap, watch the sunset or practice some deep breathing exercises.

Taking Action to Stay Positive

A diabetes diagnosis can be shocking and scary. Your automatic reaction may be to think, "I'm doomed!" But once you have time to think about the situation, you try to focus on the positive. At least now you know the situation, rather than being blissfully unaware as you continued to eat the wrong foods while your blood sugar skyrocketed.

The nice thing about this knowledge is that you can take action. And taking action can be a very effective way of dealing with challenges. Sitting around worrying or feeling sorry for yourself only makes you feel worse.

By taking action, you feel empowered and in control. What actions can you take? Here are some ideas:

- Go to the library or bookstore and get as many books about diabetes as you can find. Knowledge is power!

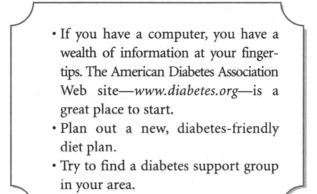

- If you have a computer, you have a wealth of information at your fingertips. The American Diabetes Association Web site—*www.diabetes.org*—is a great place to start.
- Plan out a new, diabetes-friendly diet plan.
- Try to find a diabetes support group in your area.

♆ *Think about . . .*
ways to take action

To keep myself moving and my mind focused on something positive, I will:

- Think of a family project related to diabetes that we can all do together.

- Call local schools or youth groups and offer to do a presentation on diabetes.

- Ask around about any local diabetes fundraisers or organizations, and volunteer to help.

- Think of a fun outing I can do with members of my support group—a trip to a museum, for example, or a biking trip (getting some exercise is a bonus!).

- Get a pedometer, and try and set a personal record for number of miles walked in a week.

Journey of Joy

When I was first diagnosed with diabetes in the year 2000, I was certain that diabetic medication would cure me. This, after all, was the age of technology and wonder drugs. I didn't count on the weight gain—nor, as my immune system became more compromised, was I thrilled to be diagnosed with arthritis. By spring of 2004, I dragged myself into the doctor's office with the worst upper respiratory infection of my life. Gloomily, I kept repeating to myself, *People with diabetes are six times more likely to die of the flu.* By the time I placed my foot on the doctor's scale, I was so sick that I was convinced that death would be the good news. Then I noticed my weight. I weighed in at 196 pounds! I was four pounds away from becoming my grandmother!

My doctor loaded me down with a two weeks' supply of antibiotic and a bottle of prednisone—and then he quit his practice. Now I had to search for another doctor. This was the last thing I needed! I was terrified, but in spite of my fears, my search turned out to be one of the greatest blessings of my life. Through family networking and gut-wrenching prayer, I found a soft-spoken Dutch woman a doctor who did not see my medical condition as a death sentence. She envisioned my condition as a launching pad to greater health. She was open to alternative ways of diabetes control. She was compassionate, insightful, and she was enthusiastic about my plan for exercise and a low-carb diet. "You can do it," she assured me, and I believed her.

I went home, and I really searched my heart. Do I believe that my life and my body are gifts of God? Do I believe that I have a responsibility for my own health? Do I believe that the only way I can thank God for this life is to honor his gift? Do I owe my children a mother? Do I want to grow old with the love of my life? My answer then, and now, is a resounding YES!

A year ago, I celebrated my fifty-eighth birthday by purchasing a motorized treadmill. I began a healthy, low-carb diet, including many varieties of low-carb vegetables and fruits. By the end of the first month I had worked my way from "huff-and-puff" to a half-mile, and I had lost six pounds! My taste buds became more sensitive, so that I began to notice the unique flavors of fresh foods. An apple and a couple of tablespoons of peanut butter became pure ambrosia to me. Without added sugar,

I discovered that I loved the real taste of blackberries and blueberries.

It was amazing how quickly I adapted to my new healthy lifestyle. Thankfully, I made my decision at the beginning of the low-carb movement. I have discovered delicious low-carb foods, right in my local grocery store. I could even treat myself to low-carb bread, puddings, and my personal favorite, chocolate milk. I devoted myself to reinventing my favorite recipes, creating healthier, low-carb yummies, like muffins and pancakes!

In just a few months, I was walking a mile a day on my treadmill. Naturally impatient, it was difficult for me to walk in place for an entire half-hour with only my thoughts to entertain me. Therefore, I decided to set aside that time as a time of worship. While listening to my favorite hymns, I thank God for every good thing in my life. I have been surprised to find myself also thanking him for my difficulties, which have created within me a stubborn perseverance and strength.

In the past year, I have lost nearly fifty pounds and four dress sizes, and I'm still losing! I test my blood sugar frequently during the day, especially before and after exercise. Eight months ago, I was taken off all diabetes medication, and my blood sugar, on my fifty-ninth birthday, remains happily under control. My arthritis is less painful, and I am gardening once again. My failing immune system has rejuvenated. I am fighting off infection and disease, and I have more energy than I have had in years!

I am looking forward to my future. I have a deep belief that I owe God something for my life and the love that he has given to me. My family deserves to have me in their lives, and I am worth this effort. I would not have missed this journey. It has been a journey of joy!

♥ *Jaye Lewis*

The Medical Approach

Some people will tell you diabetes is just a lifestyle issue; in other words, that it's your fault. That simply isn't true. Diabetes is a serious medical condition that requires serious treatment. Some of that can be in the form of traditional medicine.

DIABETES PILLS

Many diabetic people need to take pills to keep their condition under control. Contrary to popular misconception, these pills are not insulin. (Insulin is currently only available in injection form.)

There are several types of diabetes medication available in oral form:

- **Thiazolidinediones** help improve insulin's effectiveness. Actos and Avandia are two diabetes medications in this category.
- **Biguanides** increase insulin's ability to transport glucose into the cells. Glucophage and Glucophage XR are examples of this type of medication.
- **Sulfonylureas** make the pancreas release more insulin, thereby lowering glucose levels. Glucotrol, DiaBeta, Amaryl and Micronase are some of the medications in this category.
- **GLP-1 Analogs** are a new class of diabetic

medications called incretin mimetics (so called because they mimic the effects of GLP, a hormone produced by the intestine when food is digested). Byetta (which comes in injection form) and other drugs of this type may help patients who were unsuccessful with other diabetes medications.

Pramlintide, brand name Symlin, is another injectable sugar-lowering medication that may be given before meals.

Other types of diabetes pills include alpha-glucosidase inhibitors (such as Precose) which slow down the rise in blood glucose. There are also short-acting insulin secretagogues, such as Prandin®.

DIABETES INJECTIONS—INSULIN

Everyone with Type 1 diabetes—and some people with Type 2 diabetes—needs to take insulin shots on a daily basis. A typical person with Type 1 diabetes will take three or four insulin shots every day. There are currently several different types of insulin available, including rapid-action and long-acting varieties.

Traditionally, diabetic patients took insulin using a syringe. Today, you can also use an insulin pen. Some patients prefer using the pen, especially those with a needle phobia, because the pen looks much less scary and the needle is smaller. Also, most insulin pens come prefilled, so it's more convenient.

Where on your body will you give yourself this injection? That depends. Partly, it's personal preference, but your doctor may also have some recommendations. Abdomen and thighs are frequently used sites, but arms and buttocks may also be used. Depending on what type of insulin you are taking, your doctor may feel certain sites would be better. In certain parts of the body—for example, your thighs—insulin is absorbed more slowly. If you are taking a longer acting insulin, choosing one of these sites will cause an even longer wait before the insulin begins doing its job and there will be a longer effect.

Doctors generally recommend using the same general area every day for your injections, to keep your insulin absorption consistent.

Your doctor will help you determine the best schedule for your insulin shots. Some insulin is needed for metabolism even when you are not eating, and some is given according to your meals, so your insulin can go to work when your body is digesting the food.

Diabetic Teen Tackles Needle Phobia

At the age of sixteen, there are so many things a teenager wants to do, and staying in a hospital is usually not one of them. I had been in the hospital for almost a week, having been recently diagnosed with Type 1 diabetes and dangerously close to a diabetic hyperglycemic coma.

For the previous six months, I'd been getting more and more lethargic and losing more and more weight. My school exams were upon me, but I couldn't study—my eyes were too blurry to read any font smaller than 20 point. I eventually diagnosed myself, and my parents took me to the doctor, who told us that I was to go immediately to the hospital, otherwise I might die. Even though I was very groggy and tired, it certainly made an impact. I knew I was very sick—at five foot, four inches, I had lost over seventeen pounds in just three weeks, and that morning I had weighed only ninety-four pounds.

My first few days in the hospital passed mostly in a blur. I slept, ate, slept, ate, slept and had various educational sessions with endocrinologists and dieticians, after which—no surprise—I slept again. Partly I was exhausted, but I think I was also hiding from my new reality—that of being someone with diabetes. Once I'd digested the information that I would be on insulin injections several times a day for the rest of my life, the horror set in. I've always hated injections; they even beat spiders on my Top Five List of Very Scary Things. The nurses had up to this point been coming three times daily to give me my injections, but now it was time to do it myself.

The instructing nurse stood patiently at my bedside. She was encouraging, but was a no-nonsense woman. I knew I wouldn't be able to stall for long. Just at this point, the woman in the opposite bed started howling with pain. My ward wasn't a private one; I had four ward mates, and this woman was the chattiest. Whenever we were both awake at the same time we would talk endlessly. She had an acute kidney problem that caused "more pain than giving birth to ten kids all at once." She wailed and thrashed in agony, and doctors were crowding into the room ordering morphine.

With the noise and bustle and cries of intolerable pain in the background, I suddenly knew that I could do this. After all, here was this lovely lady, in so much pain . . . how could a lousy little injection compare? How could I be such a baby when it came to such a small amount of pain? So I took a deep breath, and with a shaky, sweaty hand, I plunged the syringe in. I survived. I could do it.

Sixteen years later, I still haven't forgotten that woman in pain who somehow made it possible for me to start injecting myself. Now, whenever I'm faced with difficulty—be it emotional or physical—I silently thank her, for letting me know it could be much, much worse.

♥ *Sonya Nicole Nikadie*

Life Anew . . .
The Tale of Type 2

O n September 29, 1998, the day before my forty-third birthday, I was diagnosed with Type 2 diabetes. I wasn't really shocked at the diagnosis; I hadn't been feeling very well for about three months. My eyesight had changed drastically in July of that year, and my eye doctor changed my prescription. The very next month, I had another change in my eyesight and went back to the eye doctor. He altered my prescription and asked me if I had diabetes. I looked at him like he was crazy. He told me that I should go to my regular physician for a checkup.

Although I considered what he told me, I didn't actually go until the end of September. By then, I was drinking massive amounts of water and eating a bag of candy a day trying to quench my cravings. I had become very dizzy and lightheaded and my vision was very blurry. When I finally went to the doctor, my sugar level was so high the blood glucose meter could not give an accurate reading. The laboratory technician told me to have a seat outside and not to leave.

Boy, the thoughts that ran through my head then. I just knew they were going to admit me to the hospital. When the doctor finally came and spoke to me, I told her that I would do whatever it took to get my sugar under control. She gave me the name and phone number of a nutritionist and a prescription for a blood glucose meter and test strips. She told me to check my blood sugar twice a day for the time being.

I went home determined to get my sugar under control and make my life better. I called the nutritionist and made an appointment. But before I could go, my eyesight began to change again and it scared me. When I called the doctor and told her, she prescribed medicine (Amaryl) for me to use temporarily until I could get straightened out. I immediately adjusted my diet and cut out all the extra sugar such as candy and cookies. I also began to read every container that I bought to see how much sugar each contained. The nutritionist taught me how to count carbohydrates and how much to eat from each food group.

I modified my diet and started working out at a local spa. I took two milligrams of Amaryl daily until I went back to see the doctor in December. My blood sugar was within the normal range. I had worked very hard to gain control of my blood sugar, and for my reward, the doctor dropped my Amaryl dose to one milligram daily. I was very happy—my goal was to control my diabetes without medication. I had been checking my blood sugar twice a day up until that point. When the doctor dropped my dosage of medicine, she also told me I only had to check my sugar once a day.

I had a follow-up visit in February of 1999 and my sugar remained at the same level it had been the previous two months. The doctor took me completely off the medicine and had me check my sugar once every four to five days. I've been back on the medicine a few times since then, but nothing I couldn't get under control.

I've done well since then. I had a checkup in September; my sugar is still within control and my hemoglobin A1C is normal. I've been completely off medication since February and feel well. I continue to watch what I eat and exercise four to five days a week. I am what you might call a "regular" at the spa.

I wanted to tell my story because a lot of people seem to think they cannot handle this disease. You can do it. It's not that hard if you use common sense. Find someone you can trust and talk to them for help. Let them be your voice until you feel ready to face it. Don't put off going to the doctor if you think something is wrong. If it is, they will let you know, and if caught early enough, you'll be fine.

I know that each and every person out there has it within them to take care of this disease. It's a lifelong process, but you don't have to suffer endlessly. I know it's hard if you're a young person, but remember, this is your life not someone else's, and you want to sustain it for as long as possible.

♥ *Karen Proctor*

Monitoring

YOUR GLUCOSE LEVELS

When you have diabetes, life sometimes seems to revolve around one magic number. Not your income or your weight, but your glucose level.

Lots of things can affect your glucose level—and unfortunately many of them (such as stress or illness) may be beyond your control. That's why it's crucial for you to pay attention to the factors you can control by eating a proper diet and taking your medication conscientiously.

YOUR KETONES

If you have diabetes (especially Type 1), it's also important to watch your ketones. These are acids in your blood. If your body is low on insulin, ketones will be present in your urine. This isn't good, as ketones are harmful to your body. This is another reason why it's important to monitor your glucose levels carefully. If your sugar levels are high, your doctor may recommend keeping a close eye out for ketone problems.

MONITORING BLOOD SUGAR AT HOME

It's important for people with diabetes to keep close tabs on their sugar levels. Some tips on checking your sugar levels:

- Your doctor will give you guidelines for when to test your blood and what your ideal glucose range is.
- Generally, you check your sugar levels first thing in the morning, before meals and at bedtime.
- There are many different types of home glucose monitors available today, ranging from basic to high-tech and fancy. Ask your doctor for advice on which monitor may be best for you. Word of mouth is also helpful—ask diabetic friends if they like a certain model best.
- Some new models have improved the process by requiring less blood or displaying results more quickly.

Painting Life by Numbers

Numbers are important.

I've learned telephone numbers, birthdates, social security numbers, driver's licenses and fax numbers. I've numbered my time, the gray hairs on my head, and use them to rate the order of my interests or the people in my life. I praise my daughter for learning her numbers and how to use them. A whole book of the Bible is dedicated to numbers.

But it wasn't until recently that I fully realized the impact of numbers in my life. After two years of not feeling well, of praying for more energy, my doctor and I began the search for a cause. I woke up in the middle of the night with a racing heart and a feeling that I was going to pass out and never wake up again. Sometimes these spells came during the day, suddenly and terrifying.

First came the blood pressure and pulse numbers to watch. Then came the cholesterol and triglyceride counts. As a result, fat content numbers and percentages were read, counted and calculated.

Then came the new numbers that detailed the level of my blood sugar. Results: high. Declaration: "Mrs. Lay, you are a diabetic."

Now I have new numbers to add to my cast of many.

I left the doctor's office afraid, confused, and frustrated that my life had just become more complicated, that the necessary act of eating and planning meals was becoming a career. I questioned God and prayed that the doctor was wrong.

But more tests showed that the doctor hadn't been wrong. I looked at my four-year-old daughter and cried. Would I live to see her children?

Numbers again. A daily sugar count and the grams of sugar in my food must come before taste or familiarity. Grocery shopping became a lesson in mathematics. My once quick excursions to the store quickly changed into lengthy reading sessions. I considered taking a lawn chair along.

After awhile, I became fairly adept at looking at the number of grams and counting, adding, dividing, then moaning or rejoicing.

On my first trip to buy groceries after learning of my diabetes, I was shocked and frustrated at the sugar content of the food and drinks I had previously enjoyed. The majority of what I picked up was returned to the counter. Too much fat. Too much sugar. Too much of both.

I became angry at the thought of the food, full of these culprits of bad health, waiting on the shelves for unsuspecting customers. Then, I became frustrated. Again I questioned God's plan for my life, wondering how taking medication and checking my blood sugar every day would fit into my busy lifestyle.

Wasn't there anything I could just enjoy, I shouted at a bottle of catsup? Anything. Something that wouldn't cause guilt, fear, or affect my health.

Then, I saw it. A can of sardines. I used to love them when I was a kid. I shook my head. There had to be something wrong with them too. I turned over the can and stared in wondrous surprise at the low fat and sugar content.

Like a girl on her wedding day staring at her new husband, my emotions took hold. I clutched the sardines and cried. It was something I liked, and I could eat it. I glanced around to make sure no one was watching my display.

As the first year has passed, I've found my attitude changing. I've met and read of others with adult-onset diabetes. I've found that it is life-changing, yet not life-disturbing unless allowed to become that way.

Friends have asked what has kept me motivated to continue walking, to stay on my diet, to lose the weight, to go on with my normal activities.

I tell them fear of complications and wanting to feel better. But, I know it's much more. It's the joy in my young daughter's eyes as we play ball in the backyard or laugh together at the amusement park. It's the times of friendship, intimacy and planning for the future with my husband. It's the conversations and good times we have with our friends. It's the satisfaction and fulfillment of seeing my writing published and of speaking to school kids.

People who've dealt with cancer in their lives or other diseases struggle to understand that they are still loved and have a place in life. I've talked with some who say that others look at them differently when they know. Then they see themselves as little more than a vessel for their illness. Yet God has given me so much more.

I am a diabetic. My mother is a diabetic and her mother before her as well. But even more, I am a wife, mother, daughter, sister, friend, writer, neighbor, speaker, Sunday School teacher, club president, teacher to my daughter, companion to my husband.

Although I carry my diabetes with me, it's only a small part of who I am. It took months to accept this, to understand that I have a full life ahead of me, the same as the day before my doctor's announcement.

I learned this from my four-year-old daughter. "Sweetheart, Mommy is . . . well, kinda sick," I explained one day when she asked why I stuck my finger every morning.

I went into a long, yet diluted explanation of my diabetes, that I couldn't eat things with sugar and that I had special medicine to take.

She listened patiently, then said, "I'm sorry." After a moment, she took my hand. "Mommy?"

"Yes?" I asked.

"But can you still play with me?"

I grabbed her in my arms and said, "You bet."

And life has gone on. And I number every blessing it brings.

♥ *Kathryn Lay*

Diabetes and Your Diet

Some important facts about the diabetes-diet connection:

You have a much higher risk of developing Type 2 or gestational diabetes if you're overweight.

It's vital that you keep your weight under control if you have diabetes. Your doctor or a nutritionist can help you prepare a diet plan that is best for you, paying careful attention to the amount of sugars and carbs. Saturated fat is a big concern, as well.

Don't be too quick to jump on the low-carb bandwagon. This is not necessarily a good approach for everyone. Your body needs *some* carbs, and some carb-containing foods, such as fruits and vegetables, are a vital part of a healthy diet.

THE DIABETES FOOD PYRAMID

The American Diabetes Association recommends using the Diabetes Food Pyramid to help maintain a healthy diet. This is slightly different than the traditional food pyramid in that the diabetes pyramid groups foods based on their carbohydrate and protein content instead of their classification as a food.

Here's a description of each group in the Diabetes Food Pyramid, along with the ADA's daily intake recommendations:

- Grains/Starches: bread, pasta, starchy vegetables, and so on. You should eat six to eleven servings per day
- Vegetables: at least three to five servings per day
- Fruit: two to four servings per day
- Milk: nonfat or low-fat varieties are preferable. You should get two to three servings per day.
- Meats: includes beef, chicken, turkey, fish and so on. Select lean cuts and keep portions small. Your target should be four to six ounces per day, spread out among meals.
- Fats: this includes sweets and alcohol. You should consume as little as possible from this group.

For more information about the Diabetes Food Pyramid and recipes for healthy meals, visit the ADA Web site at *www.diabetes.org.*

Making Healthy Eating More Fun

In the past, the term "healthy diet" conjured up images of bland-looking rice cakes with a cardboard taste. That's no longer the case. These days, there are seemingly endless varieties of healthy foods, many of which taste just as good as more fattening fare. Here are some suggestions for making it more fun to eat right:

Have a tasting party. Invite a bunch of friends over, and have everyone bring a few healthy food items—preferably new products that most of you haven't yet tasted. Let everyone sample tiny portions of each, and do your own "market research" by comparing notes on which products you liked the best.

Try the opposite approach. Invite friends over for a great meal, without alerting them in advance that everything you serve will be diabetes-friendly. Ideally, they'll like the meal (or at least most of it) and then you can reveal the truth—proving that good food can also be good for you.

Add some spice to your life in the kitchen. Take some cooking classes, or just watch some cooking shows on TV, and concentrate on finding healthy recipes with strong flavors and interesting tastes. Soon you'll be making nutritious dishes with pizzazz!

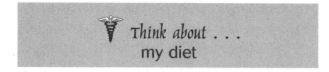

Think about . . .
my diet

Just because you've been diagnosed with diabetes
doesn't mean you're doomed to a lifetime of eating
stuff that tastes like cardboard. Obviously, if you're
accustomed to eating a box of cupcakes every day,
you'll have to lose that habit. But there are ways to
make healthy eating enjoyable.

- *Do I really know what I need to eat?* First, make
  sure you are clear as to what you should and
  shouldn't eat. You might be surprised to learn
  that some of your favorite foods are on the
  "okay" list. Study the Diabetes Food Pyramid
  and consult your doctor or nutritionist for a
  detailed diet plan.

- *What are my favorite healthy foods?* Even the
  biggest junk food junkies like at least a few
  "good for you" foods. Develop as many creative
  recipes as possible based on those healthy sta-
  ples. For help, check online recipe sites.

- *How can I avoid temptation?* If you can keep
  sugary snacks and other unhealthy foods out of
  the house completely, that's a huge help. If not,

at least keep these items somewhere out of your sight.

- Can I get my family on board? It is far easier to eat a healthy diet if everyone else in the house is doing it too. Try to enlist your family's help by getting them to join you in the quest for a healthy diet.

A Sweet Good-Bye

We never repent of having eaten too little.

THOMAS JEFFERSON

From the time he was a little boy trading his peanut-butter sandwich for some other kid's raisins, my father has loved sweets. If it had sugar in it, he wanted it. At the age of thirty, though, all those little goodies were catching up with him. He had a pot belly and a few chins to match, so one day he gave up sweets entirely. He didn't cut back; he didn't try some fad diet, eating sweets only after five o'clock on alternate Thursdays. He simply said never again. No cookies hot from the oven, no gooey brownies, no crispy and crunchy caramel corn, no velvety creamy cheesecake, no tart but smooth key lime pie: all were banished from his mouth and his table. Not so much as an after-dinner mint would cross his lips.

People thought that he'd give up after a couple of months, but it's been thirty years now, and in all that time, he hasn't indulged in even a small bite of the Christmas fudge. He's been tempted by sugar-free goodies, but long ago he decided that one low-carb brownie would lead to the real thing, and in a month or two, he'd be eating chocolate-covered peanuts by the handful.

Instead of sugar, he started jogging. At first, he ran a couple of laps around the block, but in a couple of years, he was training for marathons. He went through blisters, sore knees, chafed skin and painful arches, but he kept running. He's now run marathons in a dozen states and a couple of foreign countries, and though he's cut back to half-marathons now that he's a granddad, he still thinks that a 10-kilometer race is like a day off.

These years haven't been easy for my father. My sister and I both love to bake, and I'm sure the sight of our chocolate pecan pies, lemon tarts and banana nut cake with cream cheese frosting (my specialty) left him salivating. No matter what temptation faced him, though, thinking of what he accomplished helped him to stay strong—or maybe watching my expanding rear end was deterrent enough.

My father's sister, on the other hand, never went in much for exercise or watching her diet. We live in the South, a place where even our pies are fried, and she's more than happy to indulge in all our regional treats. Whether it's fried chicken with pan gravy, creamy squash casserole or ham biscuits, her table (and every stomach nearby) is full to bursting with good things. Every holiday she whips up big batches of fudge, divinity and macaroons, and she definitely eats her share. The last time she ran, it was to the freezer to get some extra ice cream.

My father told her gently that maybe she should eat more vegetables and less sugar. "I've never touched that stuff, and I'm not going to start now," she'd say, piling up her plate with another serving of sweet-potato pie.

A couple of months ago, my aunt called my father. She had fallen victim to the family history of diabetes. She couldn't understand why my father had no signs of it yet, even though he was several years older.

My father thought of his years of eating salad and fish rather than Lane Cake and barbecue. He thought of those thousands of miles pounding the pavement rather than pushing the remote control. Then he said that he guessed he was just lucky.

As soon as he got off the phone, he laced up his running shoes. He was going to make a happy and healthy future his own way.

♥ *Lydia Witherspoon*

A Reluctantly Reformed
Junk Food Junkie

As a young girl I heard terrible scary stories about diabetes. My paternal grandmother had diabetes; the doctors wanted to amputate her legs, but she refused and ultimately died after much suffering. Then my younger brother was diagnosed a few years ago with diabetes. I had symptoms for several years but was in denial. This was partly due to the ingrained fears I already had and partly due to the fact that I had recently been diagnosed with an autoimmune disorder. I kind of felt like life had already given me a big enough challenge, so why another one so soon?

But the time came when my doctor insisted on a three-hour glucose tolerance test. Did I forget to mention that I have terrible veins and I hate needles? Well, this test was the worst part of the whole diabetes scare. Fortunately, I have Type 2, which is controlled by oral medication and diet. Good-bye, Twinkies; good-bye, Hershey bars; good-bye, soda (I can't stand diet soda) and good-bye, cookies. My husband was watching out for me, and he wanted to know why the drawers were all filled with candy and cupcakes! The grandkids loved visiting my bedroom, where the stash of junk food was hidden. I was a junk food junkie. I had to put a stop to that. I'll admit, this diet wasn't something I rushed into with great enthusiasm. Kicking and screaming was more like it. It definitely took some getting used to.

Then I had a serious scare—and a major wake-up call—when my diabetic mother was rushed to the ER with sky-high blood sugar and had seizures for hours. I realized my mother had gotten a miracle as she survived that night, even though she had coded several times. I also realized "someone up there" was sending me a message to wake up and rearrange my priorities. Diabetes can be controlled, but it takes a bit of effort and willpower. It also helps if you focus on the added bonus of losing extra weight.

I won't lie—I still love the cupcakes. But I've grown to love fruits and other healthy stuff, too. Plus, I've discovered that sweets taste even sweeter when you save them just for special occasions.

♥ *Marcelle Kraynak*

Dining Out

If you have diabetes, that doesn't mean you have to kiss your favorite restaurants good-bye. It's very possible to enjoy a delicious dinner out while sticking fairly close to your nutritional program. Some tips:

- *Bypass the bread.* Sure, it may look innocent, but bread can be one of your biggest enemies. Bread is loaded with empty calories and tons of carbs. Just a few pieces of bread can sabotage your entire day's diet.
- *Choose desserts wisely.* We're not going to order you to give up desserts completely. We think that's unrealistic—plus you'll end up feeling resentful and deprived. But you should try to make wise choices. The dessert menu runs the gamut from healthy treats to nutrition no-no's. By selecting the smartest desserts, you'll feel like you indulged, even though you stayed on track.
- *Watch the little extras.* You know the old saying about good things coming in small packages? Well, when it comes to your diet, bad things can come in small packages, too. Those little extras like dressings, syrups and sauces can be dietary landmines. Little quantities can pack a big punch of carbs, sugar and other hidden

hazards. If you can't do without these extras completely, ask to have them on the side, so you can control how much you use.

- *Pay attention to portions.* Restaurant servings are notorious for being oversized. Don't be embarrassed to ask for the kid's version (bonus: it's often much cheaper than the adult variety). Or order an appetizer that you and a friend both like, and split it fifty-fifty.

READER/CUSTOMER CARE SURVEY

We care about your opinions! Please take a moment to fill out our online Reader Survey at **http://survey.hcibooks.com**. As a **"THANK YOU"** you will receive a **VALUABLE INSTANT COUPON** towards future book purchases as well as a **SPECIAL GIFT** available only online! Or, you may mail this card back to us and we will send you a copy of our exciting catalog with your valuable coupon inside.

First Name _____ MI. _____ Last Name _____

Address _____

State _____ Zip _____ Email _____ City _____

1. Gender
☐ Female   ☐ Male

2. Age
☐ 8 or younger
☐ 9-12   ☐ 13-16
☐ 17-20   ☐ 21-30
☐ 31+

3. Did you receive this book as a gift?
☐ Yes   ☐ No

4. Annual Household Income
☐ under $25,000
☐ $25,000 - $34,999
☐ $35,000 - $49,999
☐ $50,000 - $74,999
☐ over $75,000

5. What are the ages of the children living in your house?
☐ 0 - 14   ☐ 15+

6. Marital Status
☐ Single
☐ Married
☐ Divorced
☐ Widowed

Comments
_____
_____
_____
_____

Do you have your own Chicken Soup story that you would like to send us?
Please submit at: **www.chickensoup.com**

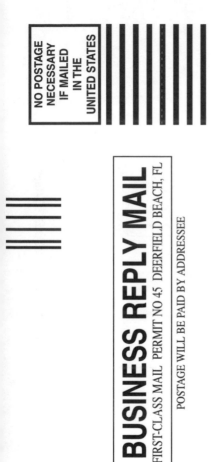

BUSINESS REPLY MAIL
FIRST-CLASS MAIL PERMIT NO 45 DEERFIELD BEACH, FL

POSTAGE WILL BE PAID BY ADDRESSEE

Chicken Soup for the Soul®
Healthy Living Series
3201 SW 15th Street
Deerfield Beach FL 33442-9875

I Want a Cookie

"I want a cookie!" Claire wriggled into her booster seat between overfull grocery bags in the backseat of the car. The bags fluttered and rattled as we drove out of the parking lot. She rummaged through the sacks, scattering apples, cereal boxes and cans of frozen orange juice.

Three weeks earlier she had begun using an insulin pump—a small device that injects insulin into the body via a tube. For two years, since Claire's diabetes diagnosis, we had measured food, measured insulin and eaten on a schedule. The pump was supposed to release us from some of the tedium that comes with diabetes, plus give Claire the freedom to eat what she wants, when she wants, without me hovering over her. But Claire wouldn't even press the pump's buttons. She would never be independent.

The plastic bags crackled. "Where are you, cookies?" Claire said in her sweet little-girl voice.

Independence meant reading nutritional labels on packaged foods, estimating the carbohydrates in all other foods, calculating her carbohydrate to insulin ratio, and entering that number into her pump. I didn't expect her to take on all these responsibilities right away, but she needed to begin. Pushing buttons with guidance seemed the logical place to start.

"Ah, ha! Can I have a cookie?"

Meeting her eyes in the rearview mirror, I saw her balancing the bag of Oreo cookies on the top of her head.

"If you punch in the numbers, you can have a cookie."

"No. You do it."

As a six-year-old, she readily recognized numbers, counted to one hundred, and could perform simple addition. With ease she pressed buttons on the television remote control to tune in her favorite cartoon show or switch from the television to the DVD player. But when we sat down for dinner and I told her the number to type into her pump for her insulin needs, she hesitated, cried and then thrust her hip, where the pump was clipped to her waistband, in my direction, her hands behind her back.

In the car, I let out a frustrated sigh. "Claire, I'm driving. I can't push the buttons from here."

"I-wan-ta-cookieee." Mournful sounds hung like a heavy mist in the backseat.

"You can *have* one. You just have to push the buttons."

I drove out of the mega-mall district and onto a stretch of road where old-growth trees waved in the breeze. The bags in the back stopped fluttering. Claire sat still. The car engine chugged rhythmically.

Parenting manuals don't discuss the intricate dependence/independence issues between a parent and child when the child has diabetes. The line between gentle prodding and pushing too hard was a fine one. We were on our own, making up rules as we went along.

From the booster seat came a small, thin, "Okay."

Oh! She said okay! "Great! Hand me the bag." I threaded my hand, palm up, between the bucket seats.

I felt the weight of the Oreo bag in my hand. I pulled it through the seats, scanned the nutritional label and calculated the amount of insulin needed for one cookie.

With care, I told her what to do. In my mind, I could see the pump in her pudgy hand, her dainty index finger poised over the select key and then the up arrow key. After delivering the last direction, the pump chirped as if to say, "well done."

"I did it! Can I have my cookie now?"

We sailed down the winding streets toward home.

"Yes. You see? I told you, you could do it."

The pump ticked out the needed insulin. She was

learning to rely on this little machine. With proper care, maintenance and direction, the pump would do its job. With time and practice, Claire would learn to take care of her health.

The car rolled up over the lip of the driveway and we were home. My hopes ran high. Independence would come, one cookie at a time.

♥ *Jennifer Angelo*

Get Moving!

You don't look good in sweats, you're not coordinated, you're out of shape . . . it's not difficult to come up with a hundred reasons not to exercise. The truth is all you need to do is set aside a little time. Exercise is important for everyone, but for people with diabetes it is especially critical. Even ten minutes three times a week can lessen your symptoms—you can work your way up to thirty minutes as your stamina improves. You don't even have to leave the house—exercising with a video in front of your TV in the privacy of your own home is just as effective as exercising outdoors or exercising at the gym.

EXERCISE CHOICES

- **Walking** is a great way to get started, especially if you haven't exercised much before. At first, don't worry about how quickly you walk. To build muscle and speed your weight loss, try walking with light hand-held weights. If you're concerned walking will put stress on your back, hips or knees, you may want to try walking in a pool.
- **Cycling,** either on a real bicycle or on a stationary machine, provides a good aerobic workout. For best results try riding up and down gentle

hills. Be sure you dial up at least some resistance on stationary machines.

- **Aerobic dance** is a great way to get fit and meet new people. Many aerobic classes incorporate weight training into their routines. Low-impact aerobics, in which one foot is always on the ground (no jumping or running in place) is safer, especially if you're new to exercise or more than a little bit overweight. Try beginners' aerobic dance videos, too.
- **Swimming** exercises your whole body and won't overstress your muscles and joints. Pushing the water away from you provides natural resistance that builds up your muscles. You can add to the resistance effect by using hand-held paddles.
- **Circuit training** with weight machines is a highly effective technique available in most gyms.

Here are some other ideas to get you started:

- Choose activities you enjoy and can fit into your daily schedule. Don't choose a morning swim routine if you hate getting up early.
- Don't worry if you miss a day or two—just do your best to make exercise a regular part of your life. Soon you'll realize you don't feel quite so good when you don't exercise!
- Find someone who will exercise with you.

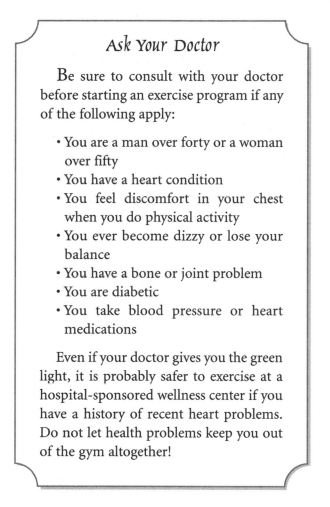

Ask Your Doctor

Be sure to consult with your doctor before starting an exercise program if any of the following apply:

- You are a man over forty or a woman over fifty
- You have a heart condition
- You feel discomfort in your chest when you do physical activity
- You ever become dizzy or lose your balance
- You have a bone or joint problem
- You are diabetic
- You take blood pressure or heart medications

Even if your doctor gives you the green light, it is probably safer to exercise at a hospital-sponsored wellness center if you have a history of recent heart problems. Do not let health problems keep you out of the gym altogether!

⚕ *Think about . . .*
ways to "sneak" exercise into my day

Instead of:	Try this:
Driving to the corner store	Walk, or ride a bike
Using the elevator	Take stairs, two at a time
Reading on the couch	Read on exercise bike
Talking idly on the phone	Do lunges while chatting
Just doing household chores	Add ankle/wrist weights

The Beltway Assassin

I received some crummy news recently: I was told I have Type 2 diabetes, which I did not have at my previous checkup six months earlier. It is caused, I am told, by being overweight. And not getting enough exercise.

Actually, the phrase isn't overweight; it's obese, which I resist. When I look at myself in the mirror, and suck myself up to my full patriarchal form, I don't see obese. I see a fantastic guy with a lifelong love affair with Wheat Thins. And if they can be called Wheat Thins after what they did to me, I should be able to sidestep obese.

Until the early seventies I was the proverbial rail. I ran, I frolicked, I burned calories instead of storing them as fat cells in case of future famine.

What happened? I got my first PC, that's what.

Oh, there were other things, like having two children and being married to an impossibly beautiful woman and buying a house and having the weight of its mortgage descend on my surprisingly unpadded shoulders. But this is about technology. I wasn't one of those guys who eat while computing, although the Pepsi Syndrome did claim a couple of keyboards early on. *The Diet Pepsi Syndrome,* he added defensively.

No, it was just so fascinating having this machine that could do whatever I told it to. I loved writing on it, and tracking submissions and managing a business. It was my friend even when it was feeble. Then when it bulked up, and the Web and e-mail arrived, I was a goner.

One day—November 12, 1994—I stopped jogging every day. I blamed it on the cold, and an arthritic knee. But the doughnut trucks kept rolling. And how I loved those chili cheese burritos at Taco Bell. So comforting, and so oozy.

It was not an overnight deal. I was not a professional pie-eating contest entrant. It was that extra drumstick here, a quaff of delicious grain beverage there. All I gained was a pound a year. But as Polonius says of his wound when Hamlet stabs him: "Tis not so deep as a well, nor so wide as a church door, but mind you 'tis enough."

Well, something's as wide as a church door. But it ain't the wound.

I know not all computer users are flabolas. But a lot are. I remember a *What's My Line* segment when I was a kid, where a not-thin gentleman signed in, and panelist Bennett Cerf—whose son truly would invent the Internet—guessed right away he was with Univac. Even then the writing was on the wall.

No, it's everyone who comes home after work, scarfs down a quick meal and retires to the serenity and intrigue of the online world. It's a virtual, twinkling, incorporeal realm. And it is groovy. But the reality is we continue to occupy non-virtual bodies, and they, like the dog that brings you the leash in his teeth, need to move periodically.

How do you know you've got a problem? My doctor put it this way: If you're sitting down, and you look down, and you can't see your belt without punching your stomach down like a batch of bread dough, by George, you've got it.

So I have to lose thirty pounds. They tell me if I do that, the diabetes will go away, and high blood sugar will no longer destroy blood vessels that feed vital nerves—like to my feet, eyes, heart and brain. The ear is shot irretrievably, but I can still save all that other neat stuff.

So here I am, your worst nightmare. I'm your mom, sans spatula. Someone with good advice and a true scary story, learning American Sign Language online and warning you to stop and think about how you're living.

I'm telling you to turn off the box, rise up from your swivel chair and go for a walk outside. *That's right,* he said cruelly, *a brisk one.*

And that sandwich protruding from your

pocket? It's time to set it free. I know it's hard. But fly away, little bird, fly away.

♥ *Mike Finley*

Healthy Relationships, Healthy Life

One common casualty of a diabetes diagnosis? Friendships and other relationships. These bonds can start to suffer if you spend too much time obsessing about your condition or making your friends feel like they're your caretakers. Some tips for keeping your relationships strong:

Feel free to ask for help, but don't overburden one person, or take advantage of their friendship.

Don't allow them—or, worse yet, force them—to be your "sugar police." If you reach for a piece of food and someone asks, "Are you sure you can have that?" just keep it light and assure them you're being conscientious of your sugar levels. Otherwise, you will inevitably begin to resent having a "babysitter." The good news: they're only concerned because they care about you—once they're reassured that you're taking your health seriously, they'll probably ease up.

Share your newfound health and nutrition knowledge with your friends—in a way that's fun, not preachy. For example, treat them to a night out at a trendy restaurant that happens to specialize in nutritious, diabetic-friendly fare. Or establish yourself as the primo salad maker of your crowd, and invite people over often to sample your healthy creations.

A Family Project

It's a great idea to involve your family in your diabetes treatment program. For one thing, having a supportive group of people around you is a huge morale booster and can help keep you motivated. Especially in the case of children, having some kind of active role in your treatment can keep them from feeling helpless. Try to think of some way to make this a fun project—by researching the amount of sugar/carbs in some of your favorite foods, or having "family fitness" adventures where you have a day filled with physical activity. A bonus: virtually all of the lifestyle recommendations for people with diabetes (staying fit, eating a healthy diet, and so on) are great for everyone in general, so your family may become healthier just by following your routine with you.

Think about . . .
my diabetes partners

▼ People who will help me live better with my diabetes: _____

_____

_____

▼ People who will hinder my ability to live well with diabetes: _____

_____

_____

▼ People I need to tell, but who I'm worried won't be supportive: _____

_____

_____

▼ My strategy for dealing with these people: _

_____

_____

_____

The Emotional Impact of Diabetes

"Just get away from me. Back off! Don't touch me." My husband's voice echoed around the restaurant. *How embarrassing!*

Their father's outburst left the children wide-eyed and bewildered. Glancing toward the table next to us, I saw questioning stares.

Although it had happened many times before, I was struggling to cope with my husband's sudden hypoglycemic reaction. For insulin pump-dependent Type 1 diabetics, blood sugar balance can be a constant battle. Some days no amount of careful planning, diet and monitoring can offset a hypoglycemic reaction.

Low blood sugar results in a number of physical and emotional symptoms: profuse sweating, trembling hands, disorientation, confusion and a feeling of panic. When Jim experiences hypoglycemia, he feels helpless and out of control and views those attempting to aid him through a cloud of paranoia and distrust. Rational thought diminishes and it becomes impossible to reason with him.

The feelings Jim experiences following a

hypoglycemic reaction can send him into an emotional tailspin. Feelings of failure, defensiveness, embarrassment, anger and defeat frequently surface. At times, the combination of emotions is so complicated it is impossible to clearly define.

Most difficult for me is the personality change. While hypoglycemia is a medical emergency, the altered personality gives the situation a surreal quality. When a person you love, and who loves you, shouts for the world to hear, "Back off, don't touch me," a wounding occurs that is difficult to heal. I understand he is speaking irrationally, yet his words hurt.

That day, as I worked to stabilize my husband's blood sugar, he became my worst enemy. As with a child refusing to take medicine, he fought my efforts to the point of becoming combative. I feared he would literally lose consciousness and fall to the floor.

Over twenty-five years of marriage, I've learned my reaction to Jim's need is my greatest responsibility. Sometimes, all I want to do is escape the situation, avoiding the panic and embarrassment of what he might say or do, but I must focus and be calm and capable.

During moments of crisis, I've learned the power of prayer. When dealing with an irrational loved one, prayer provides the comfort and courage to meet the present challenge. I am powerless in my own strength to face the situation with wisdom and calmness.

Several years ago, a hypoglycemic reaction nearly took Jim's life. The highway patrolman's flashing blue light and the sight of the mangled wreck against the guardrail are etched in my memory. Miraculously, Jim walked away from the wreckage with minimal physical damage. It was years before he allowed himself, or me, to express and deal with the emotions surrounding that night.

Ultimately, the disease affects our relationship as a couple as well as our relationships with the children. There is the tendency to deny the disease and ignore the ramifications, both present and future. It is easier to not think about potential kidney failure, amputation or blindness. It is hard to not play at "normal." But the low blood sugars, constant monitoring, wounds that take too long to heal and the bathroom counter full of all sorts of preventative medications are our reality.

Most diabetics battle depression at some point. Depression often lurks for the family as well. The disease is chronic and invasive, a never-ending part of life. Because the disease is "invisible," relatives, friends and acquaintances often see the disease as merely a nuisance. They don't understand the everydayness.

While there is usually great support in the community for individuals and families dealing with terminal illness, society remains unaware of the emotional difficulties associated with a chronic, life-threatening disease.

With diabetes some things are more doable than others—the diet, exercise and insulin pump therapy. The emotional turmoil is more difficult to confront. Only recently has my husband been able to address the anger and fear he feels and realize that in subtle ways he is often non-compliant.

Was I prepared for what lay ahead when we married? No. Did I know he would face retinal hemorrhages, temporary blindness and eye surgeries? No. Did I know we would have to work really hard to maintain emotional intimacy? No. Would I have chosen to marry him if I had known? YES!

When you love someone, you don't stop when circumstances are difficult. When the "or worse" is harder than you expected it to be, you find the good things about your relationship and savor them. You work together to discover ways to be encouraging and supportive. You make every moment count.

♥ *Candy Arrington*

Healing the Pain of a Pin Cushion

My husband and I live with a pin cushion. She's our only child and that's how she feels despite her spunky cartwheel legs and strong monkey bar arms. Her friends see a gymnast, a dancer, a kind person who loves animals and other children. I see that too, but . . .

For four years, people didn't notice the holes, the places in her tender skin where she'd been repeatedly stabbed three to six times a day. Nor did they hear the screams or witness the kicking of legs in a body too young to understand why her parents were hurting her.

Insulin injections were keeping my daughter alive. But, as her mother, how could I better nurse her wounds, the mental ones and the ones left by the needles?

At first, we covered up the pain of diabetes, those droplets of blood that dripped from her outstretched finger tip or the headaches and dizziness caused by low blood sugars. Few people saw our tears or heard the raised voices of frustration, but family life changed. We never left home without bringing an emergency kit slung over a shoulder. Like thieves we would sneak around doing glucose tests in the backseat of our car. We'd squeeze into bathroom stalls to draw up insulin into a syringe like a heroin addict. We felt dirty as though we had done something wrong. Our daughter refused to tell people about her condition for fear of being made an outcast.

We started hearing disturbing stories from other parents in the same boat.

Carly had another seizure last night. Her eyes rolled back and she started to turn blue.

I gave Donald the wrong dosage of insulin. I overheard a woman at the hospital say, "I think that little boy's dead."

Tyler didn't get off the bus. He was having a low blood sugar reaction and everyone around him thought he was sleeping. We almost lost him.

Each day I prepared my daughter's needles and wondered when another pin would drop. We were so tired. All we wanted to do was to climb out of the quicksand.

Desperate to find help, we flew to Florida in July 2003 to attend a national diabetes conference for children and their families. Over 1,500 people attended the event and, with Disney World hovering in the background, we found Tinkerbell's wand, the magic that would restore laughter to our home.

I saw how other families rose from their sorrow to make a difference in their lives. One father created *www.childrenwithdiabetes.com*, which is now one of the largest diabetes related Web sites in the world.

As a freelance writer I interviewed several celebrity role models. Adventurer Will Cross, through the two-year NovoLog Peaks and Poles Challenge, is close to becoming the first American and the first person in the world with diabetes to summit the tallest mountains on each of the seven continents and walk to the North and South poles. He credited his ongoing success to new technologies and his supportive family—both in his home and community.

"When I was diagnosed 29 years ago, managing my diabetes was a lot less convenient than it is now with the introduction of new insulin and injection pens. My mom was a strong advocate allowing and seeing that I could play sports," he said.

"My dad told me, 'Youíve got diabetes, deal with it and get on with it.' They, along with my diabetes care team, showed me that when I manage my health, I can do just about anything someone without diabetes can do."

Hamish Richardson, a member of the band Brother, told me, "You can use diabetes as an excuse to not do or be who you want to be . . . or you can find a strong spot that says 'Okay I'm different.' At some point everyone is going to have a challenge." Both reminded me that people with diabetes can do great things.

But it was a teenager, Clare Rosenfeld, who impacted me the most. She started an International Diabetes Youth Ambassador group to encourage youth to speak about their experiences and to create a better understanding of diabetes in their communities. During her speech at the conference banquet, I could feel the power of her voice stirring within me. If a teen could speak out, so could I.

I hugged my pin cushion daughter knowing that our family didn't need to hide our feelings anymore. Rather, I needed to take away the bloodstained tissue to show people the holes, the dark pits of despair that these needles can inflict upon families.

Today, our family's pain is soothed knowing that our voices can make a difference. Mothers are organizing support groups. Fathers are helping with fundraising dances and walks. Children with diabetes are lobbying governments and siblings are writing speeches about their experiences.

As Zippora Karz, a former ballerina with the New York City Ballet, reminded me, "Diabetes isn't a death sentence. At some point, you need to take a breath and say okay this isn't fair but what can I do to become the best me?"

Today our family is thankful that we climbed out of our black hole. Diabetes made us appreciate life more.

♥ *Debbie Okun Hill*

Asking for—
and Accepting—Help

Let's face it, nobody likes asking for help. And if you are the stubbornly independent type, asking for help can seem akin to failure. Well, you need to reprogram your thinking. Everyone needs help sometimes, and there is no shame in asking for help. You shouldn't hesitate to reach out to your loved ones for help—especially since, presumably, you are quick to offer help whenever they may need a hand.

People with diabetes sometimes find that they need a little extra help, mainly when they may be feeling under the weather or experiencing a diabetes-related complication.

If you're not accustomed to asking for help, this may not come naturally to you. Here are some tips that may help:

Don't be too proud to accept offers. Ideally, friends and family will offer their help before you even need to ask. They wouldn't offer if they didn't care, so don't feel like you're imposing by accepting their gesture. If friends offer to help, and there's something you need, let them know.

Spread the responsibility. Be careful not to over-burden one person by continually relying on only him or her for help. By asking each person for an occasional favor, you avoid causing any one person to burn out.

Rely on your diabetes support group. Hopefully, you have found a diabetes support group—or even just assembled an informal diabetes network consisting of friends and associates who also have the disease. You may find it easier to ask each other for help, because you all know you're in the same boat.

Communicate. People may not be aware of your needs, or may not want to offend you by assuming you need help. Often, people with diabetes (or other medical conditions) become resentful when others don't help—when in reality nobody was aware that any help was needed. Or maybe they're not sure exactly what you need. If a friend drops in to help with your housecleaning, but what you really need is a ride to the drugstore, speak up.

Be sure to reciprocate. Friends are happy to help, but nobody likes being a giver all of the time if they never get to be a "taker" once in a while. Friendship is a two-way street—to avoid looking like a user, be sure to offer your own help in return when a friend is in need.

Get Some Diabetes Buddies

Staying healthy when you have diabetes can be hard work. There are lots of lifestyle changes, daily glucose testing, medications, doctor visits and other responsibilities. It takes discipline and can sometimes be daunting. Having other people around who are facing the same challenges can be a huge help. Try and find a local diabetes support group or other organization in your area. If there's no formal group, make your own little club. Odds are, there are at least a few other people in your family or social circle who have diabetes or are at risk of developing it.

This group can be a priceless asset. You can provide each other with moral support, helpful information and a sympathetic ear. It's also much easier to motivate yourself to work out if you'll have a friend there exercising along with you. Ditto for your diet—if you have lunch with a friend who also needs to watch his or her blood sugar, it'll be easier for you to stay on track.

From the Eyes of a Sibling

I stood in the hallway and watched as my mother fussed over my brother and tended to his needs. I became more and more angry as the minutes—which seemed more like hours—ticked by. I just wanted her to look at the picture that I had colored for her. *It's as if she does not even know I exist,* I thought to myself.

"Mom, can you come see my picture now?" I said with hope. My mom turned to me in frustration. "Honey, can't you see that I am trying to give Jimmy his shot and get him dinner? His sugar is low and he needs to eat soon. I will look at your picture later."

I turned and ran to my room, slammed the door, flung myself onto my neatly made bed and began to cry. I knew that there would be no later. There never was. *It's always about Jimmy, never about me.* I quietly said to myself. *She won't come, I know it.*

I got up from my bed, wiped my tear-stained cheeks, grabbed my picture and ripped it to shreds. I then threw myself back onto my bed for more self-pity.

A few moments later, my door opened and in

came my mother. She sat down on the edge of my bed and said, "Okay, sweetie, where's that picture that you wanted to show me?"

I sat up and wiped my tears again, then looked down to where I had torn up my picture. *If it wasn't for them, my picture would still be beautiful,* I thought to myself.

I pointed her into the direction of the shreds and turned my back on her. "There's your stupid picture," I said with anger in my voice.

She left the room and returned only a moment later with tape in her hands. She sat on the floor and put every piece of my picture back together. "This is the best picture you have ever colored for me." She grabbed me up and hugged me tight. "You know, sweetie, I love you more than anything in this world. And even though I have to give a little more attention to your older brother at times, please know that I will always be here for you."

I now sit here at age thirty-seven, with two beautiful daughters of my own that I love very much. And my youngest daughter has Type 1 diabetes. With the memories that I have as a child, I prepare myself to be ready to sit with tape in hand, ready to put back together a beautiful picture that my other daughter has colored for me.

There may be only one that is sick, but both feel the pain.

♥ *Jodi Munro*

Major Complications

As the stories in this book have shown, there is no reason to be afraid of diabetes. However, you should know that diabetes can lead to more serious complications. The best solution, of course, is to be informed, be alert and be in contact with your doctor whenever the need arises.

HEART DISEASE

According to the Centers for Disease Control and Prevention, 3.5 million people with diabetes had coronary heart disease in 2003.

- Heart disease is caused by damage to the arteries, which can cause blockages and blood clots. Heart disease can be present without any symptoms.
- Heart failure is more common with people with diabetes. One common early sign of heart trouble is fluid retention, so alert your doctor if you begin experiencing swelling in your feet, legs or other parts of your body.
- Keeping your cholesterol and blood pressure within a good range can be a big step in avoiding heart disease.
- Ask your doctor if aspirin therapy is right for you.

STROKE

Stroke is another serious concern for people with diabetes. The main danger sign that you may be at risk for a stroke is high blood pressure.

KIDNEY PROBLEMS

Diabetes is the most common cause of kidney problems and kidney failure. Your doctor will suspect a possible kidney problem when protein is present in your urine. Blood sugar and blood pressure control are important. In addition to lifestyle changes, your doctor may also prescribe medication. Some blood pressure medicines provide special kidney benefits. In cases of advanced kidney damage, dialysis or a kidney transplant may be necessary.

NEUROPATHY

Diabetes may cause nerve damage. This may cause loss of sensation in your feet. Foot calluses or injuries may go unnoticed unless you check your feet daily. Proper footwear should be discussed with your health care team.

KETOACIDOSIS

Ketoacidosis (sometimes called DKA) happens when ketones in your body reach a dangerously high level. This is a serious condition that can put you in a coma or can even be fatal if not treated right away. Warning signs include a sudden major thirst and the need to urinate more frequently than usual. You may also feel nauseous or dizzy. Get medical help right away, should you suspect ketoacidosis.

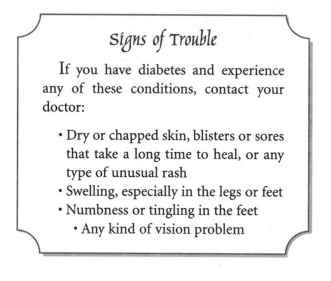

Signs of Trouble

If you have diabetes and experience any of these conditions, contact your doctor:

- Dry or chapped skin, blisters or sores that take a long time to heal, or any type of unusual rash
- Swelling, especially in the legs or feet
- Numbness or tingling in the feet
- Any kind of vision problem

♆ *Think about . . .*
ways a diabetes diagnosis
has improved my life

One good thing about a diabetes diagnosis is that it often prompts people to make positive changes in their lives. By focusing on the good things, you can maintain an upbeat attitude.

♆ Have I lost weight? If so, have I been able to buy new outfits, or fit into my "skinny" clothes that haven't fit me in years?

♆ Have I gotten into better physical shape? If so, can I do things I couldn't before, like take a long walk with the family?

♆ Did I use this experience as a wake-up call to appreciate things I took for granted, such as my health and the support of friends and family?

♆ Have I gained some new friends through my newfound support groups?

♆ Have I put my knowledge about diabetes to good use, by educating other people?

Dancing with Diabetes

Instead of waltzing into the "real world," my senior year of high school felt like a disco dance in six-inch stilettos. Why? I was diagnosed with diabetes. Thanks to high blood sugars, and all I had to learn, exhaustion reigned. Ginger Rogers, I was not.

The two-month period prior to my diagnosis, when I ate chocolate like a champion pie eater and didn't gain a pound, made my introduction to diabetes management more difficult. Imagine learning to dance the jitterbug by reading the steps in a book. The result is what my diabetes care resembled—an Energizer Bunny with a couple of screws loose.

Insulin shots hurt. My eyes-closed-hit-or-miss method of syringe injections left me bruised. Finger pricks stung. And the limited sugar diet plan from the dark side had me stumbling over my feet and ready to give up.

Then came prom night.

I spent my one and only senior prom watching blurry forms on the dance floor because my eyes were adjusting to normal levels of glucose. I'd managed to bring down the thousand-plus numbers that registered on my previous blood test, only to squint through strobe lights at the flower-decorated tables.

Despite my struggle to see, I tried to enjoy the sweet smell of roses in my prom bouquet and pretend that the delicious-smelling buffet foods were really chopped liver. That didn't work for long. Especially with the chocolate cake.

I was too depressed to dance.

But I couldn't give up either. I had my whole life ahead. So I danced anyway. Bruised toes and a ripped hoop skirt didn't stop me. I couldn't see anyone's disapproving stares so I made the best of a difficult situation and ended up enjoying myself. And I learned a valuable lesson.

Dance. Even when life hurts. It's better than the alternative.

I'm not a sidelines type of person, so after my prom night lesson, I resolved to learn all I could about diabetes. I gave myself to the dance and managed both diabetes and an active college life. After graduation I started insulin pump therapy. With the freedom from scheduled meals and boring food exchanges, I felt like doing a jig.

Then at twenty-four, I found the perfect partner and life settled into a nice slow dance. Long walks and talking until all hours of the night inspired me to take even better care of myself. I had a lot to live for. I stopped pump therapy a few months before my wedding date and I maintained hemoglobin A1C's of 6.5. Shots and finger pricks had become everyday steps. No more flinching.

Then came children.

Pregnancy with diabetes felt like a slam dance of fear. Blood sugars over 200 inspired nightmares of every conceivable complication. Brain damage. Deformity. Death. At my first doctor's appointment all I heard were the words, "You have a 40 percent chance of losing this baby if your control isn't perfect."

Perfect?

I left in tears.

When my blood sugars were up, I felt like the worst mother alive. My baby was depending on me for her very existence and I was overwhelming her little body with sugar.

Returning to pump therapy helped, but the fear of complications for my baby and myself still nipped at my heels.

I wanted to sit this dance out.

But I couldn't. So I remembered my prom lesson and danced anyway.

With each of my three pregnancies there was a little person inside that I longed to hold, to watch grow into adulthood. To do that I had to dance with diabetes and master the basic steps again. More insulin, mounting piles of test strips, and menacing fear kept me fast-stepping the entire nine months.

Even my A1C's in the 5.8 range couldn't prevent the collective gasp in the operating room when my youngest was born. She weighed eleven pounds, eight ounces. Three weeks early.

"I do believe she's the biggest baby I have ever delivered," my obstetrician said.

Years later she still is.

Her size didn't matter then and it still doesn't. She was and is a beautiful, healthy little girl. Just like her two older sisters. With their first wails, I cried tears of joy. Then when their blood sugars were normal and I could hold them, my heart danced.

I've enjoyed holding them every day since. And teaching them to dance.

My daughters haven't had to master diabetes management. I hope that's one dance they won't have to learn. But if they have to dance this dance, I know exactly what I'll teach them.

Dance. Even when life hurts. It's worth every step.

♥ *Amy Wallace*

Resources

The **American Diabetes Association** (ADA) provides lots of information about diabetes, its symptoms, treatment, meal planning and recipes, and much more.
www.diabetes.org
1-800-DIABETES

Children with Diabetes is an online community for kids with diabetes and their families.
www.childrenwithdiabetes.com

Cleveland Clinic
Resource guide provided by the Cleveland Clinic
http://www.clevelandclinic.org/socialwork/diabetes_resource_guide.htm

DiabetesNet
Diabetes information, plus a wide range of diabetes books and other products
http://www.diabetesnet.com/

Diabetes Forecast
Monthly magazine with the latest updates about
diabetes treatment and research, plus practical tips
for daily living
http://www.diabetes.org/diabetes-forecast.jsp

Juvenile Diabetes Research Foundation (JDRF)
Information and resources for people with
Type 1 diabetes.
www.jdrf.org

Who Is Jack Canfield,
Cocreator of *Chicken Soup for the Soul*®?

Jack Canfield is one of America's leading experts in the development of human potential and personal effectiveness. He is both a dynamic, entertaining speaker and a highly sought-after trainer. Jack has a wonderful ability to inform and inspire audiences toward increased levels of self-esteem and peak performance. He has authored or coauthored numerous books, including *Dare to Win, The Aladdin Factor, 100 Ways to Build Self-Concept in the Classroom, Heart at Work* and *The Power of Focus.* His latest book is *The Success Principles.*

www.jackcanfield.com

Who Is Mark Victor Hansen,
Cocreator of *Chicken Soup for the Soul*®?

In the area of human potential, no one is more respected than **Mark Victor Hansen**. For more than thirty years, Mark has focused solely on helping people from all walks of life reshape their personal vision of what's possible. His powerful messages of possibility, opportunity and action have created powerful change in thousands of organizations and millions of individuals worldwide. He is a prolific writer of bestselling books such as *The One Minute*

Millionaire, The Power of Focus, The Aladdin Factor
and *Dare to Win.*

www.markvictorhansen.com

Who Is Byron Hoogwerf, M.D.?

Dr. Hoogwerf is a native of Minnesota who
received his medical school, residency and
endocrinology fellowship training at the University
of Minnesota and the Hennepin County Medical
Center. He spent four years on the faculty of the
University of Minnesota before moving to the
Cleveland Clinic in 1985 where he is a staff physician in the Department of Endocrinology, a member of the Cardiology Prevention Clinic. He was
Program Director for the Endocrinology Fellowship
program from 1991 to 1996 and the Internal
Medicine Residency Program from 1997 to 2004.

A past president of the Diabetes Association of
Greater Cleveland, he is active with the American
Diabetes Association including past membership
on the Minnesota and Ohio affiliate boards, the
Professional Practice Committee, Chairman of the
Council on Nutritional Sciences and Metabolism,
and a member of the 1994, 2002 and 2005
Nutrition Guidelines Task Force Groups. He was a
member of the ADA National Board from 1998 to
2001, chairman of the ADA Publications Policy

Committee from 2000 to 2002 and a current member of the Physician Recognition Committee. He is a Fellow of the American College of Physicians, a member of the Endocrine Society, a charter member of AACE, a Fellow of the American College of Endocrinology and a member of the American Heart Association.

Who Is Bobbi Dempsey (writer)?

Bobbi Dempsey is a freelance writer/editor for numerous national magazines including *Parents, Family Circle, Men's Fitness, Health* and many others. She is also the author of several books on a wide variety of topics ranging from home inspections to homemade ice cream. Her Web site is *www.magazine-writer.com.*

Contributors

Jennifer Angelo is an occupational therapist as well as a freelance writer. A handful of her humorous essays have been published in Pittsburgh and Cleveland newspapers. She is currently working on a book titled, *How I Became My Daughter's Pancreas*.

Candy Arrington's publishing credits include: *The Upper Room, Encounter, Prime Years, Focus on the Family—Your Child newsletters, Advanced Christian Writer, CBN.com,* and *Writer's Digest.* She coauthored *AFTER-SHOCK: Help, Hope, and Healing in the Wake of Suicide,* judges for the *Writer's Digest* book contest, and teaches at several writers' conferences.

Harriet Cooper is a freelance humorist and essayist living in Toronto, Canada. Her humor, essays, articles, short stories and poetry have appeared in national and international newspapers, magazines, Web sites, newsletters, anthologies, radio and a coffee can. She specializes in writing about family, relationships, cats, psychology and health.

Mike Finley lives and writes in St. Paul, Minnesota. He has lost twenty-five pounds and has his glucose numbers under control.

Sally Friedman is a longtime freelance writer who has contributed to *The New York Times,* the *Philadelphia Inquirer,* the *Ladies' Home Journal* and *Family Circle.* Her works have also appeared in the *Chicken Soup* series. Sally's essays regularly appear in newspapers around the country. E-mail: *pinegander@aol.com.*

Gary Hall Jr. is a three-time Olympian, ten-time Olympic medalist and hero to millions of swimmers and diabetes patients. Since his diagnosis with type-1 diabetes in 1999, Gary has been committed to raising awareness of diabetes throughout the world. He serves as a national spokesperson for the BD Diabetes Makeover Program.

Debbie Okun Hill is a freelance writer/poet from Ontario, Canada who started writing about type 1 diabetes following her daughter's diagnosis in August 1999. In 2004 and 2005, she shared her family's story in the Canadian Diabetes Association's national holiday card campaign distributed annually to over 450,000 Canadian households.

Marcelle Kraynak is a wife, mother grandmother and great-grandmother. Marcelle is a retired nurse and founder of Silent Santa. She loves helping to make Christmas wishes come true. Her hobbies include reading and writing. E-mail Marcelle at *marcy1944@usadatanet.net.*

Kathryn Lay is a freelance writer and author and lives in Texas with her family. Her first children's novel, *Crown Me!*, was published in 2004. Check out her Web site at *www.kathrynlay.com* for news on her writing, speaking and teaching. E-mail her at *rlay15@aol.com*.

Nellie Levine is a freelance writer and has published essays, poetry and short fiction in a diverse number of publications. Her work often focuses on the family, parenting or womanhood. She lives with her husband and daughter near Smuggler's Notch, Vermont.

Jaye Lewis is an award-winning writer whose first book, *Entertaining Angels,* celebrates life from a unique perspective. Jaye is happily married and lives in southwestern Virginia. Jaye can be e-mailed at *jlewis@smyth.net*.

Jennifer Merrill, an award-winning writer, lives in West Virginia with her husband and their three bio- and step-children. A stay at home mother, she is fond of saying, "I want to have it all, I just don't want to have it all at the same time." *http://www.jmerrill.netfirms.com*.

Jodi L. Munro is married and has two wonderful daughters. She currently lives in lower Michigan working as a real estate professional and a freelance writer. In her spare time, she likes creative photography, photo enhancing/restoration, making photo/movie CD's reading and writing. She is working towards finishing her first novel. *JodiMunro@comcast.net*.

Sonya Nicole Nikadie is from Melbourne, Australia, and currently resides in British Columbia, Canada. Sonya has published several books for adults and children (under her birth name, Sonya Plowman), and also has several years' experience in magazine publishing. She is now a freelance editor and writer. To contact Sonya, e-mail *editor@distant-earth.net*.

Ava Pennington is a Bible study teacher, public speaker and former human resources director. With an MBA in management from St. John's University in New York, and a Bible Studies Certificate from Moody Bible Institute in Chicago, Ava divides her time between teaching, writing and volunteering. Contact her at *rusavapen@yahoo.com*.

Karen Proctor is a medical transcriptionist and writer who lives in Chapel Hill, North Carolina, with Reid, her husband of thirty years and her daughter, Kim.

Marci Sloane is a registered dietitian and certified diabetes educator and graduate of Columbia University. Marci manages a diabetes center, sits on several American Diabetes Association committees, teaches nutrition online and lectures to the public and healthcare professionals. Marci authored *The Diet Game: Playing for Life!*

Amy Wallace is a wife, mother of three amazing daughters, and seventeen-year veteran of diabetes. Her recent credits include contributing author in *God Answers, Mom's Prayers.* Come visit her at *http://peek-a-booicu.blog spot.com*.

Dvora Waysman is an Australian-born writer, now living in Jerusalem. She is a syndicated journalist, a teacher of creative writing and the author of nine books, the last three being *Woman of Jerusalem* (poetry and essays); *The Pomegranate Pendant,* an historical novel; and *Esther—a Jerusalem Love Story,* published by Simcha/HCI in Florida. Visit Dvora at *www.dvora waysman.com.*

Lydia Witherspoon is a writer based in south Florida. When she's not busy working, she loves long walks and lounging at the beach.